Environment, Health and Sustainable Development

Megan Landon

Open University Press

Open University Press
McGraw-Hill Education
McGraw-Hill House
Shoppenhangers Road
Maidenhead
Berkshire
England
SL6 2QL

email: enquiries@openup.co.uk
world wide web: www.openup.co.uk

and Two Penn Plaza, New York, NY 10121-2289, USA

1005019742

First published 2006

A catalogue record of this book is available from the British Library

ISBN-10: 0 335 21841 5 (pb)
ISBN-13: 978 0 335 21841 7 (pb)

Library of Congress Cataloging-in-Publication Data
CIP data applied for

Typeset by RefineCatch Limited, Bungay, Suffolk
Printed in Poland by OZGraf S.A.
www.polskabook.pl

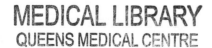

Contents

Overview of the book   xi

Section 1: Health and the environment   1

1   Introduction to health, environment and sustainable development   3
2   Environment and the development of public health   13
3   Changing pressures on health and the environment   26

Section 2: Environmental quality   39

4   Environmental quality and human activity   41
5   Energy use and sustainable development   56
6   Waste   69
7   Water and sanitation   88
8   Outdoor air pollution   106
9   The indoor environment   122

Section 3: Global issues   137

10 Global climate change and human health   139
11 The balance of ecosystems and human health   156
12 Disasters   167
13 The urban environment and health   183
14 Action at global and local levels   198

Glossary   209
Index   213

Acknowledgements

Open University Press and the London School of Hygiene & Tropical Medicine have made every effort to obtain permission from copyright holders to reproduce material in this book and to acknowledge these sources correctly. Any omissions brought to our attention will be remedied in future editions.

We would like to express our grateful thanks to the following copyright holders for granting permission to reproduce material in this book.

p. 7	Cairncross S, O'Neill D, McCoy A and Sethi D, Health, environment and the burden of disease: a guidance note, 2003 Crown copyright.
p. 91	Environmental Health Engineering in the Tropics: An introductory text, 2nd edition, Cairncross S and Feachem R (1993. Copyright John Wiley and Sons Ltd. Reproduced with permission.
pp. 170–71	Joseph Guyler Delva 'Hundreds buried in **Haiti** as flood deaths top 1,000.', 22 September 2004. Copyright (c) 2004 Reuters Limited
p. 51	D'Souza CM, 'Integrating environmental management in small industries of India,' Electronic Green Journal, Issue 14, Spring 2001 – Earthday ISSN: 1076–7975
p. 174	EM-DAT: The OFDA/CRED International Disaster Database – www.em-dat.net – Université Catholique de Louvain – Brussels – Belgium
pp. 65, 89–90	Environment and the Developing World: Principles, Policies and Management, Gupta A and Asher MG. 1998 Copyright John Wiley and Sons Ltd. Reproduced with permission.
p. 72	Eurostat, EEA on specific waste streams http://dataservice.eea.e-u.int/atlas/viewdata/viewpub.asp?id=392, June 2005
p. 89	Gleick PH, 'Basic water requirements for human activities: meeting basic needs,' Water International, 21(2): 83–92. Reprinted with permission from International Water Resources Association.
pp. 203–4	Howard G, 'Health Villages: A guide for communities and community health workers,' World Health Organization.
p. 58	IEA (international Energy Association), 2000, *http://data.iea.org/ieas-tore/defaults.asp*
p. 134	Illustration from "Smoke – the Killer in the Kitchen", 2005, ITDG website (www.itdg.org/?id=smoke_index)
p. 149	Kovats S, Wolf T and Menne B, 'Heatwave of August 2003 in Europe: provisional estimates of the impact on mortality,' 2004, Eurosurveillance Weekly, 8(11).
p. 27	Kuby M, Harner J and Gober P, Human Geography in Action, 1998, John Wiley and Sons Ltd.
pp. 47–8	Laborsta Labour Statistics Database (online). Copyright © International Labour Organisation, 2005.
p. 147	MARA website, *www.mara.org.za/mapsinfo.htm*

p. 143   © Crown copyright 2005. Published by the Met Office

p. 190   McGranahan G, et al, The Citizens at Risk: From Urban Sanitation to Sustainable Cities, 2001, Earthscan. Reprinted with Permission from James and James (Science Publishers) Ltd.

p. 142   McMichael AJ, Planetary Overload: Global environmental change and the health of the human species, 1993, Cambridge University Press. Reprinted with permission.

p. 64   Mining, Minerals and Sustainable Development: The report of the MMSD project, 2002, IIED.

p. 169   Reprinted by permission of the publisher from ENVRIONMENTAL HEALTH: REVISED EDITION, by Dade W. Moeller, p. 390, Cambridge, Mass.: Harvard University Press, Copyright © 1992, 1997 by the President and Fellow of Harvard College.

p. 84   Reprinted with permission from Waste Incineration and Public Health © 2000 by the National Academy of Sciences, courtesy of the National Academies Press, Washington, D.C.

p. 72   Source: National Statistics website: www.statistics.gov.uk. Crown copyright material is reproduced with the permission of the Controller of HMSO.

p. 144   Patz J and Kovats RS, 'Hotspot sub climate change and human health,' BMJ, 2002, 325(7372):1094–1098, amended with permission from the BMJ Publishing Group.

p. 60   Adapted from Pittman, AC Jr, Encyclopaedia of occupational health and safety, Volume III, page 76.16, table 76.4. Copyright © International Labour Organisation, 1998.

pp. 195–96   Satterthwaite D, The Earthscan reader in Sustainable Cities, 1999, Earthscan. Reprinted with Permission from James and James (Science Publishers) Ltd.

pp. 85–6   Selvam P, Community based SVM project preparations, 1994, 20th WEDC Conference Proceedings, Loughborough University. Reprinted with permission.

pp. 132–33   Smith, KR, National burden of disease in India from indoor air pollution, Proceedings of the National Academy of Sciences. Copyright (2000) National Academy of Sciences, U.S.A.

p. 163   Implementation of the United Nations Millennium Declaration: Report of the Secretary-General, 2004. United Nations

p. 22   UN Millennium Development Goals (URL: *www.un.org/ millenniumgoals*), 2005, United Nations

p. 92   Wagner EG and Lanoix JN, Excreta Disposal for Rural Areas and Small Communities. World Health Organization Monograph Series no. 39, Geneva, 1958.

p. 140   Watson RT, 'Climate Change 2001: Synthesis Report,' 2001, Intergovernmental Panel on Climate Change. Reprinted by permission of Intergovernmental Panel on Climate Change.

p. 53   Transport for a Sustainable Future: The case for Europe, Whitelegg J. 1993 © John Wiley and Sons Limited. Reproduced with permission.

pp. 126–28   Wilkinson P, Armstrong B and Landon M et al, Cold Comfort, 2001, The Policy Press. Reprinted by permission of The Policy Press.

p. 71, 74, 79 WHAT A WASTE: SOLID WASTE MANAGEMENT IN ASIA by THE WORLD BANK . Copyright 1999 by WORLD BANK. Reproduced

	with permission of WORLD BANK in the format Textbook via Copyright Clearance Center.
p. 192	World Development Report (2003) by World Bank Staff. Copyright 2002 by World Bank. Reproduced with permission of World Bank in the format Textbook via Copyright Clearance Center.
p. 131	Adapted from 'Concern for Europe's tomorrow: health and the environment in the WHO European Region', World Health Organization, 1995.
p. 101	Adapted from Guidelines for Drinking-Water Quality, 3rd edition, World Health Organization, 2004.
pp. 30–1, 36–7	"Health and Environment in Sustainable Development", World Health Organization, 1997.
p. 129	Health Principles of Housing, World Health Organization, 1989.
p. 6	Our planet, our health, World Health Organization, 1992.
p. 130	Table from "Quantifying environmental health impacts", World Health Organization, 2005. www.who.int/quantifying_ephimpacts/global/globalair/en/index.html.
p. 98	Adapted from 'Using climate to predict infectious disease outbreaks: a review,' World Health Organization, 2004.
pp. 168	"Table 11.3", from BASIC ENVIRONMENTAL HEALTH by Annalee Yassi and Tord Kjellstrom Theo de Kok, Tee Guidotti, copyright © 2001 by the World Health Organization. Used by permission of Oxford University Press, Inc.

Overview of the book

Introduction

Environmental health is part of public health concerned with assessing and understanding the impact of the environment on people and of people on the environment. This book covers three main themes – the first is an introduction to the concepts of the environment, health and sustainable development, and how these relate to one another. The second takes some specific examples of environmental quality (e.g. indoor and outdoor air pollution, water and sanitation) and explores how these are affected by human action. The third is an introduction to global environmental issues. Each chapter uses examples from low, middle and high income countries.

Why study environment, health and sustainable development?

There are several reasons why this topic should be a subject of study. These include:

1 To demonstrate the links between health, environment and sustainable development.
2 To explain equity and sustainability as central principles in environmental health.
3 To describe the environmental health risk transition in terms of differences in the pattern of risk factors and diseases within and between countries, and over time.
4 To compare examples of the impact of environmental quality including: air, water, solid waste and housing.
5 To evaluate global environmental changes in terms of health impacts and causes.

Structure of the book

This book follows the conceptual outline of the 'Environment, health and sustainable development' unit at the London School of Hygiene & Tropical Medicine. It is based on the materials presented in the lectures and seminars of the taught course, which have been adapted for distance learning.

Each chapter includes:

- an overview
- a list of learning objectives
- a list of key terms
- a range of activities

- feedback on the activities
- a summary.

The following description of the three sections and the 14 chapters will give you an idea of what you will be reading.

Health and the environment

The three chapters in this section provide an introduction to health, environment and sustainable development. Chapter 1 introduces the concepts underlying the book: health, environment and sustainable development. Each is considered in turn before an exploration of the basic relationship between environmental factors and health is undertaken in an extended exercise. Humans experience the environment as a range of physical, biological, chemical, economic, social and cultural conditions. These are interrelated and are discussed in more detail in Chapter 2, along with a short history of the rise of environmental (public) health. Chapter 3 focuses on how the environment impacts on health and how pressure is placed on the environment through human activity, including population pressure, poverty, the economy, and science and technology. The influence of the environment on human health is highlighted in low and middle income countries as they pass through the risk transition – from traditional to modern environmental threats to health. The chapter concludes with a consideration of what constitutes a healthy environment for all.

Environmental quality

This section looks at how the quality of the environment is affected by human activity and the subsequent impact on human health. A number of topics will be explored in more detail using high, middle and low income country examples, including industry, energy, water and sanitation, outdoor air pollution, the indoor environment and waste.

As countries develop, there is increasing industrialization and this has consequences for the environment and health through air, water and soil pollution, as well as waste disposal. Improving economies and rising incomes have led to an increased reliance on transport which is a major contributor to urban air pollution and traffic accidents. These issues are explored in Chapter 4. In Chapter 5, the effects of the three most common methods of generating electricity – fossil fuels, nuclear power and hydroelectric power – are considered in turn. The consideration of the sustainability of energy use is then discussed along with an introduction to renewable sources of energy. Chapter 6 considers the sustainability of different methods of waste disposal from re-use to disposal in landfill or incineration. Chapter 7 explores the relationship of water and sanitation to health. Outdoor air pollution is a significant environmental health problem in high, middle and low income countries and is discussed in Chapter 8. There are many sources and types of air pollution, each of which have different health effects. You then consider how the effects of air pollution can be studied and used to estimate the burden of disease as well as to aid in setting standards and managing air quality. As individuals, we spend most of our time indoors. Chapter 9 introduces you to the hazards of the indoor environment and concentrates on two main examples: the effect of cold homes and the burden of indoor air pollution from biomass fuels in developing countries.

Global issues

Global environmental health issues are considered in this section and the question of how sustainable development has been planned and implemented at global, national and local levels is explored. The chapters concentrate on the effects of global climate change, biodiversity, urbanization, disasters and policy issues.

Climate change appears to be a largely human-induced phenomenon. Chapter 10 covers the history, research and policy responses to this global event. The uncertainties in making estimates of the effects of climate change are explored and the role of sustainable development and equity are considered.

Chapter 11 considers ozone depletion and loss of biodiversity. While it is not possible to estimate with certainty the ultimate effects of the ecological damage caused by development, agriculture and industrialization, the ensuing loss of bio-diversity already has had a profound impact on the world's ecosystems. Chapter 12 discusses the environmental, health and economic costs of natural and man-made disasters. In the past 20 years, three million deaths have been caused by natural disasters alone. You also consider the role of planning for disaster prevention and relief. In Chapter 13 you will study the environmental health issues associated with urbanization, how they affect different populations within cities and how cities might be designed for the optimal health of their inhabitants. Chapter 14 looks at how local initiatives and grassroots movements can affect policy and also directly affect health and the environment. This chapter also provides a brief overview of international policy making and how this can influence the environment and health. It explores some Local Agenda 21 initiatives and finally looks at whether it will be possible to live sustainably in the future.

Acknowledgements

The author would like to thank the contributors past and present, involved in the course taught at LSHTM, for providing lecture notes and references as a basis for the book, specifically Sari Kovats, Araceli Busby, Martine Vrijheid, Paul Wilkinson, Ben Armstrong, Pete Kolsky, Sandy Cairncross, Shakoor Hajat, Virginia Berridge, Peter Baxter, David Sattherthwaite and Gordon McGranahan.

Thanks also to the external reviewer, Tony Gattrell, Lancaster University, for very helpful comments and Deirdre Byrne and Rosalind Raine for editorial guidance.

SECTION I

Health and the environment

Introduction to health, environment and sustainable development

Overview

Wherever people live and work is called their environment. The environment encompasses people's surroundings and the circumstances relating to their surroundings, so it includes physical, biological, social and cultural factors. People constantly interact with their environment; it helps shape their lives, and it affects their health. The aim of this chapter is to encourage thinking about how environmental health is relevant to you and your local area. Much of the chapter will be taken up by activities which will encourage you to examine your own environment in some detail.

Learning objectives

By the end of this chapter, you will be better able to:

- describe the general relationship between the environment and people's health
- understand the relationship between human activities, human health and sustainable development
- describe specific relationships between environment and health in your local area

Key terms

Environment Physical, biological, social and cultural conditions affecting people's lives and the growth of plants and animals.

Health State of physical, mental and social well-being and not merely the absence of disease or infirmity.

Sustainable development Meeting the needs of the present generation without compromising the ability of future generations to meet their needs.

Health, environment and development

The quality of the environment and the nature of any economic developments taking place are major determinants of the health of people in that environment. However, environmental health issues have not traditionally been seen as a priority

in policy making, or in developmental planning. This is despite the fact that biological agents in the environment such as mosquitoes, parasites and water-borne
bacterial pathogens are involved in the world's most significant health problems.
These factors are responsible for the illness and premature death of millions of
people (often infants and children) in the developing world, from causes such as
malaria, intestinal parasites and diarrhoeal disease. In addition, chemicals such as
pesticides and cleaning agents, and physical hazards in the home, the workplace
and the natural environment are responsible for millions of additional illnesses,
injuries and deaths. Health and the environment are not independent entities;
they are influenced by external driving forces such as population pressure and
poverty. If the world's peoples are to achieve good health, then individuals,
governments and other agencies must learn to balance the interaction between
human activities and the environment. In order to achieve this in a manageable
way, two important criteria must be met:

- Economic development must meet people's needs;
- Ecological sustainability must be achieved; this means ensuring that natural
  resources can be sustained for present and future use without being irreparably
  damaged or destroyed.

To achieve these goals, action is required on the local, national and global level
by individuals and through cooperation between governmental and non-
governmental agencies. As you read the book you will find examples of the interaction of health, the environment and sustainable development. You will also
see how individuals and professional groups can work together to tackle these
key issues.

The relationship between health and the environment varies in countries at different stages of development. For example, childhood deaths are far lower in high
income countries such as the UK in comparison to low income countries such as
Tanzania, and are largely related to traffic accidents. One of the main environmental features associated with this is road traffic, which both increases the
incidence of accidents and also contributes to air pollution. Pollution may be
responsible for exacerbating asthmatic illness. The types of illness that affect the
child population of Tanzania relate mainly to the difficulty of ensuring supplies of
clean water and the observance of hygienic food handling practices.

Adult deaths in the UK are largely the result of a relatively affluent lifestyle – where
people indulge in too much food and take too little exercise. Adult health in
Tanzania is subject to the same problems that cause childhood illness there –
insufficient fresh water and poor quality food – as well as the widespread incidence
of malaria-carrying mosquitoes and HIV. Tanzania, and countries like it, are also
facing increasing pressures on health such as those described for the UK. This
phenomenon is known as the risk transition and will be expanded upon later in the
book.

Defining the key issues

This book aims to explore the relationships between health, environment and sustainable development. You will find that there are a number of different definitions
of these terms, depending on the perspective of the author. The definitions of

health, environmental health and sustainable development that follow will be used throughout the book.

You will note that these are formal definitions, from such agencies as the WHO and various other United Nations (UN) bodies. It has only been within the past two decades or so that the alarm has sounded at an international level about the effects of environmental deterioration and its consequences for future generations in terms of human health and well-being. The international bodies, represented by the WHO and the UN in particular, have been very active in trying to develop ways to measure environmental dangers to health. There have been a number of international efforts to address issues concerning the environment and health, culminating in a series of world conferences and declarations.

Health

The WHO definition of health is that it is a state of complete physical, mental and social well-being and not merely the absence of disease or infirmity (WHO 1948). According to WHO, the conditions required for health not only include the availability of resources to meet basic human needs and provide protection from all environmental hazards, but also require a sense of security and well-being. If the environment in which you work or live is deficient in some way, this can lead to both physical and psychological problems. Health is no longer seen as being solely the responsibility of doctors, nurses and other medical personnel, but now is also the responsibility of individuals, households, communities, governments and multinational agencies. These groups have the knowledge and power to make changes in their environment and living conditions, and therefore can affect the health of the population at large.

Environmental health

WHO defines environmental health as those aspects of human health, including quality of life, that are determined by physical, biological, social and psycho-social factors in the environment. It also refers to the theory and practice of assessing, correcting, controlling and preventing these factors in the environment that potentially can adversely affect the health of present and future generations (WHO 1993).

✎ Activity 1.1

You have read the WHO definition of environmental health which suggests that physical, biological and social factors of the environment act on health. All human activity has environmental and health consequences. List some human activities that will affect health through their effect on the physical and biological environment.

Ↄ **Feedback**

The WHO definition of environmental health highlights the connection between the state of the environment and the health experiences of individuals and communities. The relationship between human activities and the environment has the potential to either impair or improve health. Figure 1.1 gives an example of the relationship between human activities, health and the physical and biological environment. The environment can be improved by human activity, for instance, by draining mosquito breeding sites in marshland or by improving housing. Human activity can just as easily impair health, by releasing toxic chemicals into the atmosphere and changing the physical environment. Some environmental agents are responsible for damage to health without human intervention, for instance, ultraviolet light from the sun, leading to the development of skin cancers; or a lack of minerals such as iodine or selenium in soil and foodstuffs leading to nutritional disorders. In these instances, human activity can mitigate the effects of the environmental agents through the use of technology, nutritional supplements or education.

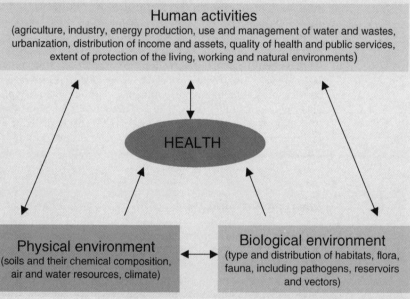

Figure 1.1 Interaction between human activities and the physical and biological environment
Source: Adapted from WHO (1992)

Global burden of environmentally related disease

The role of the environment on the burden of disease is significant; the environment has been implicated in 21 per cent of the overall burden of disease world-wide. Most of this burden falls on developing countries.

Figure 1.2 shows a breakdown of the global burden of environmentally related disease. Note the large burden of disease from diarrhoea (28 per cent); in developing countries, 1.7 million children die from diarrhoea associated with inadequate water supplies. You will read more about this in Chapter 7. The second largest health burden is acute respiratory disease; this is mostly associated with poor indoor air quality, and is discussed further in Chapter 9.

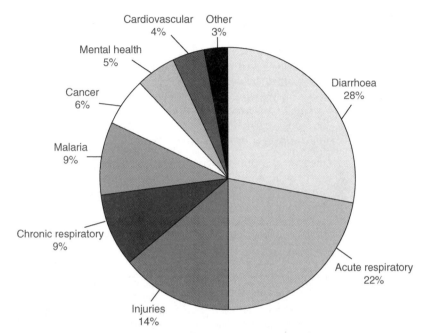

Figure 1.2 Breakdown of the global burden of environmentally related disease
Source: Cairncross et al. (2003)

Sustainable development

The World Commission on Environment and Development define sustainable development as 'meeting the needs of the present generation without compromising the ability of future generations to meet their needs' (World Commission on Environment and Development 1987). These needs include food, work, shelter and health care for all the population and they must be provided in a manner that prejudices none of them and preserves the environment and its resources.

Throughout our history, humans have interacted with the environment and freely used natural resources. It is only now that we are beginning to understand that this is no longer possible and that there are long-term consequences that can result from unrestricted use and abuse of the environment. It is this imbalance that the principles of sustainable development aim to address.

Sustainable development is also about addressing equity within the present generation. It is often the poorest groups in society who are most exposed to environmental hazards, including dangerous working conditions and restricted access to adequate and safe food and water. In addition, low-quality housing is often situated in the most polluted areas, such as contaminated land, near roads and industrial plants. The importance of this has been enshrined as part of the United Nations Universal Declaration of Human Rights: 'all people have the right to a standard of living adequate for the health and well-being of themselves and their family, including food, clothing, housing, health care and the necessary social services' (UN 1948). It is only relatively recently, however, that this declaration has been translated into action that will ensure these rights for present and future generations. A number of international meetings have been held to discuss ways forward. At the 1992 Earth Summit in Rio de Janeiro, Brazil, a number of principles relating to an integrated approach to the environment, health and sustainable development were agreed upon, along with a plan for future action. The first principle is that 'human beings are at the centre of concerns for sustainable development. They are entitled to a healthy and productive life in harmony with nature' (UNCED 1992). There will be more on the Earth Summit and follow-up meetings in Chapters 2 and 14.

The Earth Summit recognized that nature and human activity are often in conflict with one another. One of the key messages to come out of the summit was that the principle of respect for nature and the control of environmental degradation should guide human activities in order to balance the potential conflict between health and the environment. The only exception to this principle is when there is a conflict with the Declaration of Human Rights.

Activity 1.2

You have now been introduced to the definitions of health, the environment and sustainable development, as used in this book. This activity aims for you to bring the concepts together, to summarize your findings and then extend your thinking further. Use these concepts to answer the questions below:

1 What are the relationships between human activities, human health and sustainable development?
2 Can you think of the differences in the patterns of health and disease between low, middle and high income countries? What are the reasons for these differences?
3 Can you think of any differences between men and women in their relationship with the environment? What is the role of women in sustainable development?

Feedback

In order to make long-term progress and improve health and lifestyle, it is important to take the basic concerns of environment, health and sustainable development seriously. For example, it is difficult to make progress on the economic growth of a community if the water supply is inadequate for essential needs. Likewise, economic development and social growth will be impeded if communities are living in squatter camps on the urban fringe, subjected to environmental degradation and its subsequent health effects.

1 The relationship was spelt out at the 1992 Earth Summit, where it was noted that human activities are compromised by ill health and degradation of the environment.

Development cannot be sustained where water supplies are unsafe and where the waste products of human industry are allowed to pollute the environment. In these circumstances, no safeguards are being applied against communicable disease.

2 Both infant and adult mortality is much higher in low than in high income countries. There are a number of environmental factors that account for these discrepancies, including a lack of safe water supplies and sanitation, overcrowding, squalid urban conditions and the inability to vaccinate against childhood illnesses. There will be more on these issues later in the book.

3 There is a difference in the impact of the sexes upon the environment and health. Women are more vulnerable to environmental hazards because they are closely involved with the factors impacting upon basic living conditions – housing, sanitation and the provision of food and drinking water. They are also less represented in any political institutions that might consider the means of alleviating them. The impact of the environment on women is covered more fully in later chapters on water, sanitation and air pollution.

 Activity 1.3

Before moving on to examine environmental health in more depth, it is important to provide a background for your studies and show their relevance to everyday life. The best way to do this is to start with something that is familiar, so this activity requires you to think about the local area in which *you* live or work. What is it about your environment that might affect your health or that of other members of your community's?

1 Find or draw a map of your local area. Go for a walk and mark up on the map any aspects of the outdoor environment that you consider important for health.
2 How could the environmental features that you have identified affect the health of the community?
3 The WHO definition of environmental health takes account of human, physical and biological factors in the environment. Make notes on the human activities, and the physical and biological environment in your local area that may affect human health.

 Feedback

1 Your map could include the location of:

• water pipes
• sewage works
• street drains
• chimneys – domestic and commercial
• locations where food is sold
• traffic areas – roads and railway lines
• residential areas, including different housing types
• animal housing such as kennels or stables
• factories
• agricultural areas

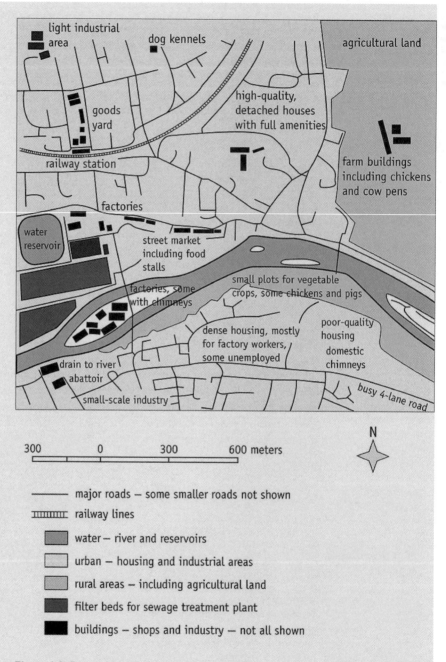

Figure 1.3 Environmental features of 'Ordinaryville'

2 A map of a fictional area called 'Ordinaryville' (Figure 1.3) is provided to illustrate the environmental features that should be taken into account when considering the effect of the environment on human health. In Ordinaryville, the wind usually comes from the west. This blows the factory emissions onto the dense and poor-quality housing. The abattoir and the island factories discharge waste directly into the river, as does the sewage treatment works. There is, however, a water treatment plant that operates efficiently to supply fresh water to the area.

Some of the roads are very busy, leading to possible problems with air pollution and traffic accidents. Animals are kept near to human dwellings, with the potential to spread infectious disease. Some of the housing is of poor quality – this could exacerbate the spread of any infectious diseases resulting from the poor quality of the plumbing or its absence. Respiratory illness may be a consequence of poor air quality. The number of road traffic accidents may be high, due to the poor level of road repair.

Some of the potential environmental problems depend on the quality of, and adherence to, local regulations concerning the housing of animals, food storage and service and industrial processes.

There are other things that could be stated about this town and its amenities, and you may have identified other important factors in your own environment.

3 You may have included some of the following points:

Human activities
- agricultural activities. These might include the types of crops grown; the machinery and fertilizers used; the extent to which crops are sold locally or exported; and government policies concerning assistance to local farmers, or crop subsidies
- industrial activities. These could indicate heavy and light manufacturing industries and the provision of water and waste facilities. This also encompasses local policies on pollution and working condition regulations and the identification of local and remote markets

Physical environment
- for agricultural regions, this would include the nature of the soil; the amount of annual rainfall and water availability and average seasonal temperatures
- for urban or industrial areas, water availability and climate might also be relevant, as well as waste provision, population characteristics and housing conditions

Biological environment
- indigenous animals and plants which are harmful to human health. For example, the malaria mosquito, or if you are in a built-up area, rats may be a problem. In rural areas, farm animals may be subject to particular parasites.

Summary

This chapter introduced the definitions of health, environment and sustainable development. By now it should be apparent that the environment plays a crucial role in the health of individuals and communities. The importance of sustainable development was also discussed. The cornerstone of sustainable development is the belief that everyone in the community should have access to a safe environment for health – and this needs to include future generations.

References

Cairncross S, O'Neill D, McCoy A and Sethi D (2003) *Health, Environment and the Burden of Disease: A Guidance Note*. London: DFID.

UNCED (1992) United Nations Conference on Environment and Development (UNCED), Rio de Janeiro: http://www.un.org/esa/sustdev/documents/UNCED_Docs.htm

United Nations (1948) *Universal Declaration of Human Rights*. New York: UN.

WHO (1948) WHO definition of health: http://www.who.int/about/definition/en/. Accessed 20 August 2004.

WHO (1992) *Our Planet, Our Health*. Geneva: WHO.

WHO (1993) *Global Strategy: Health, Environment and Development: Approaches to Drafting Country-wide Strategies for Human Well-being under Agenda 21*. Geneva: WHO.

World Commission on Environment and Development (1987) *Report to United Nations General Assembly* (A/RES/42/187), 11 December.

Further reading

McMichael AJ (2001) *Human Frontiers, Environments and Disease*. Cambridge: Cambridge University Press.

United Nations Environment Program: http://www.UNEP.org/

UN Division for Sustainable Development: http://www.un.org/esa/sustdev/

World Health Organization (WHO): http://www.who.int/

WHO (1992) *World Development Report 1992: Development and the Environment*. Oxford: Oxford University Press.

WHO (2000) *World Health Report 2000: Health Systems, Improving Performance*. Geneva: WHO.

WHO (2002) *The World Health Report 2002 Reducing Risks, Promoting Healthy Life*. Geneva: WHO.

2 Environment and the development of public health

Overview

Recent improvements in the health of urban, industrial populations owe more to social and environmental improvements and dietary changes than to medical treatments. This makes the study of issues surrounding environmental health all the more relevant. Now that you have identified environmental factors that may affect health in your own area, you will look at environmental health from a historical and then a global perspective in this chapter.

Learning objectives

By the end of this chapter, you will be better able to:

- explain environmental health in a historical context with respect to changes in technology, economic development and social organization
- describe the basic requirements of a healthy environment

Key terms

Climate change A statistically significant variation in either the mean state of the climate or in its measurable variability, persisting for an extended period (typically decades or longer).

Ecosystem A functioning, interacting system of living organisms in relation to their physical, chemical and biological environment.

Ecology The scientific study of the relationship between organisms and their environment.

Equitable development Development that is based upon the principles of equity.

Equity Fairness, defined in terms of equality of opportunity, provision, use or outcome.

Exposure The degree to which a person is subject to a given risk factor.

Industrial revolution The use of new sources of energy from fossil fuels and the employment of new technology in the development of manufacturing industry and agricultural production.

Precautionary principle A principle that advocates the use of prudent social policy in the absence of empirical evidence in an attempt to solve a problem.

Vector An organism, such as an insect, that transmits a pathogen from one host to another.

Health risks and the environment – historical considerations

To understand the relationship between the environment and health in modern society, it is useful to put these relationships into a historical context. The realization that there is a connection between health and the environment has developed slowly over time.

It is obvious that human beings are part of the world's ecosystem. An ecosystem is an interacting system of organisms and their surrounding physical, biological and chemical environment. Unlike the other parts of the ecosystem, however, humans have also evolved culturally and now have the unique ability to shape and control their environment, rather than be entirely shaped by it. Some changes have been beneficial, such as improved housing, food and water supply; others are harmful, such as air and water pollution, or potentially catastrophic, such as the capacity for nuclear war.

Technology and scientific development have brought advances in health care and birth control to large sections of the world's population. Many diseases that once were fatal or serious have now been eradicated or brought under control. In contrast, the peoples of the developed world are now faced with diseases of affluence such as cardiovascular disease and cancer.

As we have seen, biological, chemical, and physical hazards to the environment have been synonymous with human development throughout our history. Industrial pollution is not a new problem – even in ancient times, sites of production and manufacture were contaminated by pollutants. For example, lead contamination is still found in proximity to old metal smelters, and the offensive smell and heavy water pollution found near tanneries has for centuries necessitated official restrictions on where they can be sited. When the scale of industry was small, contamination was often restricted to the immediate vicinity, meaning that the occupational health and safety of those workers directly involved in production was the most significant environmental and health issue. So, whereas traditional risks affected only the local environment and inhabitants, the environmental damage associated with modern industry is more widespread. The way in which human activity now affects a wider region is part of the 'risk transition' that will be discussed in more detail in Chapter 3.

Understanding the relationship between health and the environment

There are many theories concerning the relationship between disease and the environment. In the past, diseases were attributed to meteorological events such as changes in the seasons, storms and eclipses. Many societies associated disease with bad, corrupt or polluted air from corpses, swamps, marshes and other sources. There are variations among different cultures regarding the specific environmental influences on disease that are important, but many societies have recognized that there is some kind of relationship between the two (Howe 1997). For example, Zulus believe that the people in any particular region are adjusted to their surroundings, but should they go to a completely different region they would become ill, not being adapted to the new atmospheric and environment conditions

(Ngubane 1977). Moving to a new area may subject the migrant to new diseases or to different strains of diseases such as malaria.

The way that a society views the relationship between disease and the environment will affect the way that it is able to deal with health promotion initiatives. For instance, if a community believes that dengue fever (an insect-borne disease) is caused by atmospheric conditions such as bad air, it will be difficult to convince them that removing standing water in which insects can breed is an essential action for disease eradication. It is important for the health practitioner to understand not only the theory and practice of environmental health, but also the cultural and social context in which it is to be used.

The environment and the development of public health policies

From ancient Greek times, Hippocratic ideas about air, water and place stressed the crucial role of the environment on health outcomes, but perceived the environment as a feature to be passively accepted (Glacken 1967). By the sixteenth and seventeenth centuries, however, the existence of a connection between health and the environment had become generally recognized. Good air and the elimination of foul smells were felt to be particularly important, and a healthy environment was thought to produce healthy food and drink. For many, the earth was regarded as an almost animate body that needed care and attention.

By the eighteenth century, the idea that the environment could be modified was well developed in Western societies. This led to active intervention; this was a time of great land drainage schemes in the east of England to create more agricultural land, as well as selective animal and crop breeding and attempts to promote soil fertility.

The Industrial Revolution

The Industrial Revolution began in Britain (c.1760) making it the first country to suffer the consequences of large-scale industrial pollution. Mass production led to the employment of thousands of new workers in the wage-earning class. These workers became consumers themselves, necessitating an increase in production; the profits were reinvested in further industrial expansion and the capitalist cycle of production began.

The Industrial Revolution dramatically altered the relationship between economic activity and the environment. By 1800, industrial pollution had been identified as a serious issue. This was largely due to the energy requirements of iron industries and led to both local and, eventually, more widespread pollution.

Although industrial pollution was considered a serious problem in Britain in the Victorian era (1837–1901), it was not given a high priority. Social issues such as child labour, poverty, alcohol and drug abuse, welfare services, corruption and prostitution were considered more serious and were related to the urbanization that accompanied industrialization. Communicable diseases and unsafe water supplies were the main health concerns, and coordinated responses for dealing with them were developing.

Sanitary conditions considered

In 1834, the Poor Law Amendment Act was passed in Britain; it established the Poor Law Commission – a group of government-appointed individuals whose role was to inspect and promote the care of poor people. They had to ensure that local authorities administered relief to the poor, and provided buildings to house the destitute. Previously this work, if done at all, was undertaken by church and charitable groups. One of the foci for the Poor Law Commissioners was sanitary conditions, as illustrated in the extract below which was published by the Poor Law Commission in 1842.

Report of an Inquiry into the Sanitary Conditions of the Labouring Population of Great Britain

First, as to the extent and operation of the evils which are the subject of this inquiry:

That the various forms of epidemic, endemic, and other disease caused, or aggravated, or propagated chiefly amongst the labouring classes by atmospheric impurities produced by decomposing animal and vegetable substances, by damp and filth, and close and overcrowded dwellings prevail amongst the population in every part of the kingdom, whether dwelling in separate houses, in rural villages, in small towns, in the larger towns – as they have been found to prevail in the lowest districts of the metropolis.

... That such disease, wherever its attacks are frequent, is always found in connexion with the physical circumstances above specified, and that where those circumstances are removed by drainage, proper cleansing, better ventilation, and other means of diminishing atmospheric impurity, the frequency and intensity of such disease is abated; and where the removal of the noxious agencies appears to be complete, such disease almost entirely disappears.

... That the formation of all habits of cleanliness is obstructed by defective supplies of water.

... That the annual loss of life from filth and bad ventilation are greater than the loss from death or wounds in any wars in which the country has been engaged in modern times.

... That, measuring the loss of working ability amongst large classes by the instances of gain, even from incomplete arrangements for the removal of noxious influences from places of work or from abodes, that this loss cannot be less than eight or ten years.

... That the ravages of epidemics and other diseases do not diminish but tend to increase the pressure of population.

Secondly. As to the means by which the present sanitary condition of the labouring classes may be improved:–

The primary and most important measures, and at the same time the most practicable, and within the recognized province of public administration, are drainage, the removal of all refuse of habitations, streets, and roads, and the improvement of the supplies of water.

... That the expense of public drainage, of supplies of water laid on in houses, and of means of improved cleansing would be a pecuniary gain, by diminishing the existing charges attendant on sickness and premature mortality.

... And that the removal of noxious physical circumstances, and the promotion of civic, household, and personal cleanliness, are necessary to the improvement of the moral condition of the population; for that sound morality and refinement in manners and health are not long found co-existent with filthy habits amongst any class of the community.

The report's authors realized that there were health problems associated with poor hygiene. They offered solutions before they had an understanding of how disease was transmitted. They were advocating the use of what is now known as the precautionary principle. This principle advocates the use of prudent social policy in the absence of empirical evidence, and in more recent times has been championed by environmental campaigners in particular as the best way to deal with environmental issues such as ozone depletion in the stratosphere. Waiting for scientific or other evidence before taking action would possibly lead to an exacerbated situation.

Public health in the late nineteenth century

The first law specifically dealing with public health, the Public Health Act, was passed by the British Parliament in 1848. It concentrated on environmental factors such as clean water and health hazards related to infectious diseases. The boroughs (local authorities) assumed responsibility for drainage, water supplies, paving and the removal of 'nuisances'. A Central Board of Health was also established. The effects of industrial pollution were largely overlooked at this time because the government was more interested in protecting the rights of the factory owners. The economic theory of the time argued that unconstrained economic growth would benefit all levels of society and maximal profits would attract further investment. The 'traditional' environmental risks such as clean water and sanitation provision seemed more pressing than any unknown dangers from new industry or manufacturing processes. There was no accompanying scientific assessment to address the issue of exposure to chemical pollution and its effects on public health. Understanding the causes of infectious disease helped to strengthen the public health laws.

Until the late nineteenth century, the causes of plague, fever and pestilence were still unknown. Odours and miasmas (emanations) were still considered the agents responsible just as the ancient Greeks had done. Slowly other theories were put forth including the 'germ theory' and Louis Pasteur (1822–95) and Robert Koch (1843–1920) finally were able to prove the existence of germs, and how they reproduced and caused disease. By the end of the nineteenth century, the transmission of disease via insect vectors was also understood. This knowledge meant that new ways could be found to combat disease.

The first half of the nineteenth century saw Britain establish the posts of Medical Officer of Health and a Factory Inspectorate. Sanitary investigations were instigated, and statistics were collected. Statisticians were able to use their skills to demonstrate class and regional inequalities in health. As European colonialism spread to Africa and Asia, so too did the public health message, and environmental health officers formed part of the colonial administration in many countries. The legacy of this movement is still seen today.

The rise of environmental awareness

In the later part of the nineteenth century, there was a growing awareness of the importance of the environment. Part of this awareness was a growing interest in the natural sciences, heightened by public interest in the work of Charles Darwin (1809–82), Gosse (1810–88) and many other naturalists and writers. Interest was also strong in the Romanticism of nature by poets such as Wordsworth (1705–1850), Schiller (1759–1805) and Keats (1795–1821). Nature and Romanticism were also important movements in the fields of painting, novels and music. By 1860, both the USA and Britain had passed laws aimed at protecting the environment. In Britain, the Alkali Act (1863) was aimed at enforcing reductions in hydrogen chloride (HCl) emissions during alkali production. In 1864, the US Congress passed a bill for the Preservation of Yosemite as a National Park. Around this time, possibly the first environmental campaigning group – the 'Commons, Open Spaces and Footpath Preservation Society' – was formed in England (Gupta and Asher, 1998). Early environmental movements tended to be led by professionals such as foresters, who were interested in either the preservation or management of land and resources. For example, the Sierra Club is the USA's oldest, largest and most influential grassroots environmental organization and was founded in 1892 with 182 charter members. The inaugural president of the club was John Muir, who was active in forestry as were many of the original members. The first conservation campaign was an effort to defeat a proposed reduction in the boundaries of Yosemite National Park on the rationale that, 'Everybody needs beauty as well as bread, places to play in and pray in, where nature may heal and give strength to body and soul alike' (John Muir 1912). The Sierra Club's mission statement was:

1 Explore, enjoy and protect the wild places of the earth.
2 Practise and promote the responsible use of the earth's ecosystems and resources.
3 Educate and enlist humanity to protect and restore the quality of the natural and human environment.
4 Use all lawful means to carry out these objectives (Sierra Club 2005).

In the 1960s, the Sierra Club underwent a resurgence in popularity as a result of the concerns over environmental degradation.

This management of the environment could also lead to ecological destruction; for example, British colonial powers in India felled the forests for their timber and replaced them with other species for commercial development. Local management techniques had previously worked well and meant a constant supply of timber with far less environmental degradation. The colonial management techniques led to a reduction of species and problems with soil erosion and water runoff.

As the twentieth century progressed, there were rapid changes in the technology associated with industrial applications. At the same time, a growth in consumer demand led to huge increases in the volume of hazardous materials and resultant pollution. Concern for the environment became more fragmented – the focus of public health had shifted to 'lifestyle' issues such as diet and exercise, rather than the environment. This trend continued until increasing levels of industrial pollution caused a massive public outcry in the 1960s and the 1970s in many parts of the world.

In her bestselling book *The Silent Spring* (1962), Rachel Carson detailed some of the dangers that pesticides could hold for the environment and human health. The book heightened the public's awareness of alternative ways of viewing human health in relation to the environment. There was also increasing concern over the effects of testing of atomic weapons, coupled with the occurrence of environmentally damaging disasters. Extensive publicity was given to the grounding of the tanker *Torrey Canyon* which spilled 34,986,000 gallons of crude oil on the west coast of England in 1967. These events were associated with a swelling of the membership of traditional organizations such as the Sierra Club, along with the rise of many new environmental organizations such as Greenpeace (2005).

 ## Greenpeace

When the last tree is cut, the last river poisoned, and the last fish dead, we will discover that we can't eat money . . .

Greenpeace is an independent, campaigning organisation that uses non-violent, creative confrontation to expose global environmental problems, and force solutions for a green and peaceful future. Greenpeace's goal is to ensure the ability of the Earth to nurture life in all its diversity.

Greenpeace has been campaigning against environmental degradation since 1971 when a small boat of volunteers and journalists sailed into Amchitka, an area north of Alaska where the US Government was conducting underground nuclear tests. Greenpeace promotes open, informed debate about society's environmental choices. They use research, lobbying, and quiet diplomacy to pursue their goals, as well as high-profile, non-violent conflict to raise the level and quality of public debate.

As a global organisation, Greenpeace focuses on the most crucial worldwide threats to the planet's biodiversity and environment. They campaign to: stop climate change, protect ancient forests, save the oceans, stop whaling, say no to genetic engineering, stop the nuclear threat, eliminate toxic chemicals, and encourage sustainable trade.

Concerns about the environment and sustainable development have continued to bring together individuals, groups and nations. There are now many 'grassroots' and international non-governmental organizations (NGOs) working on environmental issues. There is still widespread disagreement about environmental priorities, particularly with respect to global environmental issues and equity.

Has environmentalism had its day?

In the 1960s and the 1970s, the environmental movements made huge progress in lobbying for clean air, clean water and the preservation of many wilderness areas. The perception of major threats to the environment has now changed from local to global (at least in high income countries). Environmentalists and many of their critics agree that there has been inadequate progress to deal with global warming, particularly in the USA. Public concern has not been as engaged on this issue as it was with earlier successful environmental campaigns, such as vehicle emission controls or access to clean water. There also appears to be little political will to deal with global warming issues, and so decision makers have not had to confront the need for fundamental changes. In *The Death of Environmentalism* (2004), Shellenberger and Nordhaus argue that the focus of the environmental movement is too narrow and that it is not able to animate national debate. The 'solutions' put forward (for example, using low emission vehicles or energy-efficient light-bulbs) are neither inspiring nor on a large enough scale, and are unlikely to be successful.

Pope (2004) counters this argument by suggesting that environmentalism is still working and can be as effective as it has been in the past. The solution is not to kill off the movement, but to find ways to engage the public and policy makers on the issues. One of the problems is that opinions in the United States are moving to the political right, and environmental campaigners, who tend to have liberal attitudes, are unlikely to fully engage with a (neo-)conservative public. This is one of the reasons why there is a call for different approach. Shellenberger and Nordhaus argue that the answer to tackling global warming lies in selling the *solution* to the problem, rather than focusing on the problem itself. Today's public and politicians are most concerned about immediate and local issues such as jobs and a thriving economy, rather than the 'environment'. The solution may be support for an economy based upon new energies, not reliant on fossil fuels. This approach would mean less air pollution, more jobs and less dependence on the Middle East for oil. Critics consider that investment in this strategy is a better use of available resources than the traditional approach of environmentalists.

International agreement on the environment

The 1972 Stockholm Conference was planned as an international forum to discuss the problems of pollution. However, the agenda was extended to focus on the environment and development. There was consensus that it was necessary to preserve natural habitats and produce a sustained improvement in living conditions for all. A declaration was drawn up by high income, as well as developing nations, with an emphasis on solving environmental problems, but without ignoring social, economic and developmental factors. This has been recognized as the first move towards the idea of sustainable development and that responsibility for the state of the environment falls upon individuals as well as governments.

The increase in the number of environmental disasters and continuing concern about environmental and health issues led to a further meeting in Rio de Janeiro in 1992 (see Chapter 1). The UN Conference on the Human Environment (sometimes known as the Earth Summit) led many national governments to introduce new legislation curbing industrial pollution. In the United States, the Environmental Protection Agency (EPA) developed a range of successful, voluntary efforts to reduce or eliminate waste at the outset of the manufacturing and service cycles. Actions such as these meant a substantial reduction in the total amount of industrial pollution, despite the decline in environmental activism. The conference reaffirmed the Stockholm principles and committed 118 countries to Agenda 21 (Agenda for the 21st Century). The broad aims of Agenda 21 are to meet the challenges of global warming, pollution, biodiversity and the inter-related social problems of poverty, health and population through environmental restoration, preservation and social development (UN 1992).

The first recognition of a truly international environmental problem was the increasing hole in the stratospheric ozone layer above the Antarctic, brought about by the release of chlorofluorocarbons ('CFCs'), into the atmosphere; there is more detail on this in Chapter 11.

At the time of the Earth Summit, the international community agreed that action against climate change induced by greenhouse gas emissions was required, even if the consequences in terms of global warming were unclear. Chapter 10 considers this in more detail.

Current environmental concerns

The increasing rates of economic growth in low and middle income countries and rising world population levels have introduced a new factor into the environmental equation. Previously, most industrial production (and associated pollution) had occurred in high income countries, while in low and middle income countries, the effects of industrial pollution tended to be small-scale and localized. The rapid rise in the demand for goods in low and middle income countries has resulted in a huge increase in production and trading. Industrial production in low and middle income countries has relied on expedient, cheaper technologies and there has been little control of effluent and emissions levels. The potential for environmental problems are clear.

The divide between high and middle or low income countries in terms of environmental health priorities has become an important area of debate. The industrialized, high income countries (largely situated in the northern hemisphere) have come to realize the long-term significance of the impact of human activity on the environment. This is most apparent in the issues surrounding climate change. For progress to be made in this area, the high income nations require the cooperation of the low and middle income countries. The poorer countries (which tend to lie south of the equator) are more concerned with immediate social and environmental threats such as poverty and access to water and sanitation. Low and middle income countries may also have additional problems to contend with, related to internal conflicts and wars. These may be partially the result of rapid population growth and be tied up with social and economic factors found in these countries.

Millennium Development Goals

In September 2000, world leaders attended a United Nations Millennium Summit in New York. At this meeting, they united in their determination to achieve peace and set decent standards of living for all. To achieve these targets they agreed to work towards a set of time-bound and measurable goals. The goals focused on: reducing poverty; illiteracy; hunger; lack of education; gender inequality; improving child and maternal mortality rates; preventing disease and reducing environmental degradation. These goals now form the centre of the global political agenda, and are called the Millennium Development Goals (MDGs). The summit's Millennium Declaration included a range of commitments for all countries concerning human rights, good governance and democracy.

Table 2.1 Millennium Development Goals

	Development goal	Means
1	Eradicate extreme poverty and hunger	Reduce by half the proportion of people living on less than a dollar a day (refers to US $)
		Reduce by half the proportion of people who suffer from hunger
2	Achieve universal primary education	Ensure that all boys and girls complete a full course of primary schooling
3	Promote gender equality and empower women	Eliminate gender disparity in primary and secondary education preferably by 2005, and at all levels by 2015
4	Reduce child mortality	Reduce by two-thirds the mortality rate among children under five
5	Improve maternal health	Reduce by three-quarters the maternal mortality ratio
6	Combat HIV/AIDS, malaria and other diseases	Halt and begin to reverse the spread of HIV/AIDS
		Halt and begin to reverse the incidence of malaria and other major diseases
7	Ensure environmental sustainability	Integrate the principles of sustainable development into country policies and programmes; reverse loss of environmental resources
		Reduce by half the proportion of people without sustainable access to safe drinking water
		Achieve significant improvement in lives of at least 100 million slum dwellers, by 2020
8	Develop a global partnership for development	Develop further an open trading and financial system that is rule-based, predictable and non-discriminatory. Includes a commitment to good governance, development and poverty reduction – nationally and internationally
		Address the least developed countries' special needs. This includes tariff- and quota-free access for their exports; enhanced debt relief for heavily indebted poor countries; cancellation of official bilateral debt; and more generous official development assistance for countries committed to poverty reduction
		Address the special needs of landlocked and small island developing states
		Deal comprehensively with developing countries' debt problems through national and international measures to make debt sustainable in the long term
		In cooperation with the developing countries, develop decent and productive work for youth
		In cooperation with pharmaceutical companies, provide access to affordable essential drugs in developing countries
		In cooperation with the private sector, make available the benefits of new technologies – especially information and communication technologies

Source: UN, Millennium Goals

The eight goals laid out in the Millennium Declaration (Table 2.1) were reaffirmed at subsequent meetings in Monterrey, USA, and Johannesburg, South Africa, and were specifically designed to require a commitment by the rich countries to relieve debt, increase aid and allow fair access to markets for the poorer nations. The responsibility for achieving these goals lies not only with the rich countries; the poor countries are accountable for their own actions and are expected to take the steps required to undertake policy reform, and strengthen governance in order to achieve development.

Basic requirements for a healthy environment

You have been introduced to the definitions of environment, health and sustainable development as used by the international community. You have considered the local environment in your *own* area and the historical background to the growing concern over industrial pollution and *global* environmental issues. It is now useful to consider what the basic requirements for a healthy environment might be. This creates a starting point for policy making at a local and global level that can ensure equity for all.

 Activity 2.1

Write down a list of aspects of the environment that you think are basic requirements for health and sustainable development.

 Feedback

Understanding what constitutes a good environment for health helps us to make changes and improve health. The list below is one suggested by the World Health Organization (WHO):

- clean air
- safe and sufficient water
- adequate and safe food
- safe and peaceful settlements
- stable global environment

Sustainable development

Sustainable development is closely allied with the provision of an environment that supports and promotes health. You have already considered how the connection between health and the environment was established. This can be no longer seen as a local and small-scale issue; the effects of the environment on health are now apparent on a larger, global scale and are not confined to one point in time. As new threats to the environment and health emerge, or old threats re-emerge, new ways of using and distributing resources and protecting the environment must be considered.

Activity 2.2

Take the list of the basic requirements for health that you drew up in Activity 2.1 a stage further, and consider how the environment and the principles of sustainable development might be used to support health.

 Feedback

The WHO (1992) advanced a range of suggestions to support the requirements for healthy living through sustainable development:

- analysing the role of local environmental factors on the health development of a community
- encouraging an enabling and promotional approach to health issues, as well as simply protecting health
- creating health equity within a community
- acknowledging the importance of sustainable development as a health issue
- enhancing people's understanding of the environment in a broad sense
- promoting the active and genuine encouragement of people's participation and involvement

Understanding the different environments within a community and how they relate to health is the first step. Engaging with the community by including stakeholders in decision making on environmental and health issues promotes the ideas of sustainable development. It also demonstrates support for healthy living and sustainable development by encouraging equity in health in the community; for example, through the provision of clean water or safe housing for all members of the community.

Summary

The principles of sustainable development balance the population's entitlement to a healthy life with a consideration of the impact of economic growth upon the environment. This is becoming increasingly important as the scale of environmental problems become apparent – from the local to the global. Historically, societies have approached the relationship between environment and health in various ways. Our understanding of environmental impact upon health has changed dramatically since the Hippocratic ideas of air, water, and place; we now have a scientific understanding of ecosystems and the impact of human activity on the environment. With the rise of the importance of public health organizations and the burgeoning environmental movement came recognition of the impact that the environment has on human health. It can be argued that progress has been made in curtailing potential damage to the environment, however, much remains to be done, particularly as the concept of global economic development grows. The current challenge for professionals, politicians, communities, and environmentalists is how to deal with global climate change and its impact upon the environment and health in the long term. There are political tensions in the poorer low and middle income countries that still require urgent attention, as well as important local environmental concerns. The Millennium Goals have helped to focus international attention on improving our health and environment through sustainable development and cooperation.

References

Carson RL (1962) *The Silent Spring*. London: Hamish Hamilton.

Glacken C (1967) *Traces on the Rhodian Shore: Nature and Culture in Western Thought from Ancient Times to the End of the Eighteenth Century*. Berkeley, CA: University of California Press.

Greenpeace (2005) www.greenpeace.org. Accessed 20 January 2005.

Gupta A and Asher M (1998) *Environment and the Developing World*. Chichester: John Wiley & Sons, Ltd.

Howe GM (1997) *People, Environment, Disease and Death: A Medical Geography of Britain throughout the Ages*. Cardiff: University of Wales Press.

Ngubane H (1977) *Body and Mind in Zulu medicine: an ethnography of health and disease in Nyusu-Zulu thought and practice*. London: Academic Press.

Poor Law Commissioners (1842) *Report on an Inquiry into the Sanitary Conditions of the Labouring Population of Great Britain*. London.

Pope C (2004) http://www.sierraclub.org/pressroom/messages/2004december_pope.asp. Accessed 22 February 2005.

Shellenberger M and Nordhaus T (2004) *The Death of Environmentalism: Global Warming Politics in a Post-Environmental World*. www.breakthrough.org. Accessed 20 February 2005.

Sierra Club (2005) http://www.sierraclub.org/inside/. Accessed 20 February 2005.

United Nations (1992) Report of the United Nations Conference on Environment and Development: http://www.un.org/esa/sustdev/documents/UNCED_Docs.htm. Accessed 10 August 2004.

United Nations (2000) 55/2. United Nations Millennium Declaration September 2000: http://www.un.org/millennium/declaration/ares552e.pdf

United Nations Millennium Goals: http://www.un.org/millenniumgoals/. Accessed 10 May 2004.

WHO (1992) *Our Planet, Our Health*. Geneva: WHO.

Further reading

Environmental activism: http://www.globalstewards.org/

Environmental History Timeline: http://www.radford.edu/~wkovarik/envhist/index.html

Kriebel D, Tickner J, Epstein P et al. (2001) The precautionary principle in environmental science. *Environmental Health Perspectives* 109(9): 871–5.

Smith KR, Corvalan CF and Kjellstrom T (1999) How much global ill health is attributable to environmental factors? *Epidemiology* 10(5): 573–84.

3 | Changing pressures on health and the environment

Overview

The influences of the environment on health are not straightforward. In this chapter you will be introduced to those underlying social and economic conditions that influence the effects of the environment upon health. There are a number of different environmental hazards and risks posed to health and these can be classified in different ways. When looking at these hazards and risks and evaluating their impact upon populations and social development, it is important to appreciate the transition in risk type from traditional to modern.

Learning objectives

By the end of this chapter, you will be better able to:

- **give examples of the social and economic conditions that can adversely affect health**
- **state the difference between hazard and risk**
- **explain the process of risk transition**
- **critically discuss the positive and negative impacts of driving forces on health and the environment**

Key terms

Driving forces Factors that create the circumstances in which environmental health conditions develop or are diverted.

Hazard A factor or exposure that may adversely affect health.

Risk The probability that an event will occur.

Risk transition The process by which societies move from exposure to traditional hazards to exposure to modern hazards.

Human activity and the environment

The ways in which humans change and manipulate their environment influence the interaction between the environment and health. To discuss this further we need an understanding of those factors termed 'human driving forces' (WHO 1997). These are underlying, human-induced changes in social and economic

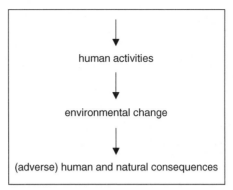

Figure 3.1 Driving forces of environmental change
Source: Adapted from Kuby et al. (1998)

conditions that can influence human activities such as industry and the provision and use of services and household consumption. In turn, these cause environmental change via the use of energy and redistribution of materials and by direct biological manipulation. These can lead to adverse human and natural consequences such as air pollution; loss of habitat for indigenous peoples; climatic change and loss of biodiversity (Figure 3.1).

Looking at Figure 3.1, the first and clearly most influential link in this chain is that of 'human driving forces'. Human activity affects environmental health, either positively or negatively. In order to fully understand this process, it is necessary to investigate the pressure that leads to human activities, thus allowing informed policy and decision making on environmental health issues. This can then lead to a situation where sustainable development can take place, and where adverse environmental changes are minimized.

The main components of those 'human driving forces' are listed below and the next part of this chapter will focus upon some of these:

- population and urbanization
- poverty and inequity (inequity relates to factors that are unequal *and* unfair. Some factors are unequal but unavoidable, e.g. genetic predispositions to illness, and so are not considered to be inequitable. Other factors are unequal and avoidable, e.g. variations in the supply of health care. These factors are considered to be inequitable.)
- technological and scientific development
- political and economic systems
- cultural values.

✎ Activity 3.1

Table 3.1 contains a list of the human driving factors that were introduced above. For each, give an example of how the factor has an important influence upon environment and health in *your* country. The first one has already been completed for a low income country.

Table 3.1 Human driving factors

Factor	Influence
population and urbanization	No comprehensive family planning strategy; unchecked migration from rural to urban areas
poverty and inequity	
technological and scientific development	
political and economic systems	
cultural values	

 Feedback

The answers you have given will be specific to your own country; there are no right or wrong responses. For illustrative purposes, possible answers relevant to a low income country have been inserted in Table 3.2.

Table 3.2 Human driving factors (completed)

Factor	Influence
population and urbanization	No comprehensive family planning strategy; unchecked migration from rural to urban areas
poverty and inequity	Uneven wealth distribution. The very wealthy have access to good sanitation services and the poor have no sanitation services
technological and scientific development	Use of solar panels to provide electricity in urban areas; support for local manufacture of pharmaceuticals
political and economic systems	Government moving towards democracy; money is still controlled by an elite few
cultural values	Belief in local medical model

Are there any other factors that you consider have a significant influence on environmental health in your country? One possible example might be an increase in industrial manufacture.

Population and urbanization

In 2004 the world's population was 6.4 billion people; this represented more than a doubling of the population over the past 40 years, and this rapid population growth is continuing. The global average family now has three children per woman. This has reduced from six per woman although this decline is less apparent in low income countries (UNFPA 2004). Low and middle income countries will be responsible for 96 per cent of the population growth, while the populations in both Europe and North America are declining, manifesting ageing populations and falling family sizes (Figure 3.2). It is not just the impact of population growth itself upon the environment that is important, but also the population structure and its

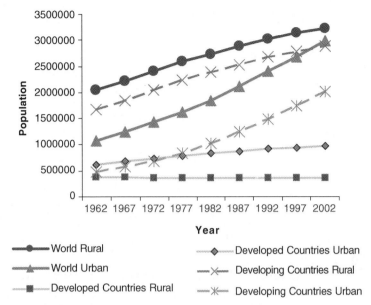

Figure 3.2 World population trends
Source: UNFPA (2004)

migration. As might reasonably be anticipated, wealthier nations have a far greater impact upon the environment than the new populations in the low and middle income world (Sarre and Blunden 1996). During any time of population increase, greater demands on the environment will take place through depletion of natural resources, combined with an increase in industrial development. As an example of this, the People's Republic of China has seen a levelling off of population growth, yet consumption is increasing rapidly at eight times the rate. This increase in consumption is due to an improvement in living standards and an increase in the economy's overall quality and efficiency (EIA 2005).

Population pressures are closely associated with the effects of urbanization. Since 1962, the urban population has increased from 1 billion to 3 billion, most of this in low and middle income countries (Table 3.3). Some 67 per cent of urban dwellers now live in low and middle income countries. In 1962, the urban population of low and middle income countries was 23 per cent of that in 2002. This is the result of a huge population growth, combined with a large migration of the population to urban areas and their fringes while they sought economic advantages and a better life. The results of these population changes have been to place severe pressures on the environment for the provision of housing, food and water. Increased population density leads to increased industrial activity and greater resource depletion. This has damaging implications for health, particularly in the poorer countries, where exploitation of the environment rather than conservation is the focus in survival. Urbanization is covered in more detail in Chapter 13.

Table 3.3 Changes in world urban and rural populations

		1962		2002	
		Population (1000s)	% of world population	Population (1000s)	% of world population
world	Total	3 140 795		6 224 988	
	Rural	2 057 107	65.5	3 233 565	51.9
	Urban	1 083 688	34.5	2 991 423	48.1
high income countries	Total	993 753	31.6	1 325 038	21.3
	Rural	381 248	12.1	351 716	5.7
	Urban	612 505	19.5	973 322	15.6
low and middle income countries	Total	2 147 042	68.4	4 899 950	78.7
	Rural	1 675 859	53.4	2 881 849	46.3
	Urban	471 183	15.0	2 018 101	32.4

Source: UNFPA (2004)

Poverty and inequalities in access to basic human needs

Inequalities in health by socioeconomic group, geographical area, gender and race or ethnicity are a significant driving force in the interaction between health and the environment. The extract below from WHO (1997) provides examples of variations in health across these social groups. The term 'inequity' used in the extract refers to factors that are both unequal and unfair.

 Examples of inequity in health by socioeconomic group, geographical area, gender and race/ethnicity

Socioeconomic group

- Life expectancy at birth of the most disadvantaged group in Mexico is 20 years less than that of its most affluent group.
- Adults in São Paulo Brazil in the late 1980s had mortality rates that were two to three times higher if they worked in a non-professional rather than a professional job.
- In Bolivia most public spending on health goes towards care for people belonging to the upper two income quintiles, although these groups already have the best health status.
- Disparities in health between rich and poor are also apparent within developed countries, although they are usually smaller; wealthy groups have the most concentrated medical attention, eat better, and can afford to live in environmentally clean and disaster-free areas.

Geographical area

- In Nigeria the average life expectancy in one region, Borno, is only 40 years, 18 less than the Bendel region.
- Although only 39 per cent of the population of the Côte d'Ivoire lives in cities, at least 80 per cent of the country's health expenditure is directed towards urban areas.
- In Lima, Peru, the infant mortality rate is 50 per 1000 births, while in some rural areas it is as high as 150 per 1000 births.

Gender

- A study in India showed the female infants were almost twice as likely to die by the age of 2 as were males, and concluded that the most likely explanation was the different behaviours of families towards male and female children, not biological differences.
- Another report concluded that the death of one out of every 6 female infants in India, Bangladesh and Pakistan was due to neglect and discrimination.
- Studies in Bangladesh found that boys under 5 years of age were given 16 per cent more food than girls the same age. Additionally, evidence is mounting that adolescent and adult women may not receive an appropriate proportion of available food within the family.

Race/ethnicity

- In Guatemala, poverty and malnutrition during the 1980s was much higher among indigenous children that non-indigenous children.
- In 1990 in South Africa death rates for non-white men were double those of white men, and more than four times as much money was spent on health care for whites than for blacks.

The most severe environmental health problems tend to affect those countries and individuals who lack access to economic resources. Stark contrasts in levels of economic affluence and health exist between nations. 2.8 billion people live on less than $2(US) a day, 1.1 billion do not have adequate access to safe drinking water and 2.4 billion lack basic sanitation (UNFPA 2004). Meanwhile just 1.7 billion (mostly in high income countries) are responsible for most of the world's energy, meat and paper consumption, as well as car driving. The groups living in absolute poverty (sometimes measured as living on less than $1(US) a day) are those who lack access to basic human needs such as food; safe drinking water; sanitation facilities; health; shelter; education; employment and health care and include a high proportion of women; children; refugees and other displaced persons (WHO 1996).

In recognition of this situation, the Millennium Declaration was signed by 189 nations in 2000. It set out eight goals to be met by 2015, with the aim of improving the living conditions for all humanity. You have already read about the development of these goals in Chapter 1; they are highly relevant in attempting to change the driving forces that impact on the environment. The first goal is to eradicate extreme poverty and hunger. The next two are directly concerned with alleviating poverty by achieving universal primary education and the empowering of women. The promotion of sustainable development is a further goal and those remaining are related directly to health outcomes. The progress toward these goals is being monitored and can be accessed on the UN website: www.undp.org/mdg

Progress has already been made towards eradicating poverty; in 1990, 17.1 per cent of the population in countries other than those termed as 'high income' had less than $1 a day purchasing power parity (PPP); by 2001 that figure had fallen to 14 per cent.

Technological and scientific development

Along with the massive rise in population growth in the past 200 years, there have been considerable advances in our understanding of the world we live in and our ability to control some aspects of it. Thus, science and technology have become significant influences on human health and the environment. Many economists tie population, consumption and technology together to describe their relative impacts on the environment:

$$I = PAT \text{ (Impact = Population} \times \text{Affluence} \times \text{Technology)}$$

In high income countries, scientific and technological advances have made significant contributions to the economy. Such advances allow more efficient agricultural methods and bring about improvements in industrial production, health care, environmental conditions and the promotion of human development. However, they are not all positive influences, as they allow the development of inefficient technologies and the production of pollution and waste products. As populations grow and consumption increases, the use of technology to create greater efficiencies in energy production and industrial processes becomes increasingly important.

Indigenous cultures have tended to integrate technological advances with their environmental context, allowing the full benefits of advancement with minimum environmental degradation. In contrast, the arrival in a society of new technologies which have been developed elsewhere will not always result in the overall advancement of social conditions. As an example, there are many new technologies available to increase agricultural output which can have potentially negative impacts, such as the overuse of pesticides and/or land degradation. The high costs of these products for individual small farmers may lead to an aggregation of agricultural land and the loss of livelihood. To best improve the economy and to protect the environment, technology should be adapted and not simply transferred; in other words, the technology must be appropriate and adapted for the environment for which it is intended.

Industrial processes and hazardous waste products are regularly transferred between countries. In the past there have been concerns that when these 'dirty technologies' are banned in one country, they are simply moved to another. International agreements, such as the Basel Convention on the movement of hazardous waste (1989), have been put in place to regulate this trade. As already discussed, the transfer of industrial technologies from high income to low and middle income nations can have negative effects, however, the converse is also true; as new, more efficient and less polluting technologies and manufacturing processes are produced, low and middle income countries can take advantage of them. For example, the manufacture of efficient, compact, fluorescent light-bulbs through joint ventures between Chinese and Japanese companies (UNFPA 2004).

Information and communication technology (ICT) has spread rapidly throughout the world and is allowing new economic ventures in high, middle and low income countries. The spread of ICTs allows societies to access information and communicate efficiently and effectively; this may be associated with the growth of democracy, and social participation. Such access to information is relevant even in those communities where little or no basic resources or infrastructure such as water or roads exist. For example, in Peru small-scale agricultural producers in Cajamarca province have been able to use computers to access a customized database that contains details of locally appropriate technology, trade and business issues. An Internet link provides opportunities to gain information on subjects including better crop production and processing methods. Most of the province's inhabitants live in rural communities and remote access points have been established to serve these people. The project was set up to test how new information and communication technologies (ICTs) can be used by small-scale producers to improve their livelihoods and reduce poverty in the area (Intermediate Technology Development Group 2004).

ICTs allow small communities to participate in global markets and can increase productivity and development by removing some of the barriers to participation, allowing these countries to engage in sustainable development. Technology can be used to support the goals of sustainable development. Policy makers and decision makers need to be informed as to how this can happen and support further research.

Activity 3.2

List positive and negative influences of scientific and technological developments on environmental health.

Feedback

Positive influences include more efficient crop production, 'cleaner' industrial processes and opportunities for remote communities to learn about agricultural innovations using the Internet.

Negative influences include loss of livelihood through the inappropriate application of agricultural methods leading to land degradation and dumping of waste in poor environments.

Technological developments will have a key role to play in achieving a balance between health and the environment and are essential if the goals of sustainable development are to be realized.

Economic development

Economic growth does not always equate with improved health and conditions for all. It is often those who already have economic power who benefit the most. Economic and sustainable development can be used to reduce poverty and improve health and the environment. For example, women in Zimbabwe are involved in a microfinance scheme where small loans and financial advice are advanced to traders, manufacturers, or service providers. This allows an increase in economic stability and allows the participants greater financial capacity to deal with health problems for them or their family members.

Economic development traditionally starts at the level of subsistence agriculture, and moves to agricultural business, industrial development and the service sector. Each of these broad economies is associated with different health and environmental outcomes.

Trade development

There are positive and negative consequences for the environment from the development of trade. For example, trade in timber from tropical forests has been shown to be unsustainable and there are now moves to regulate this trade. One response to concern about trade in tropical timber is the promotion by some companies of sales of managed, sustainable timber from high income countries.

Liberalization of trade and multilateral trade agreements are beginning to benefit both high and middle or low income countries. There are international agreements in place to facilitate free trade without barriers being imposed by particular parties, however, there is still a danger of the trade of hazardous waste (from rich to poor countries) and the use of unregulated, cheap manufacturing processes that damage health and the environment. In these cases, business practices aimed at reducing costs (sometimes used by powerful international companies) can conflict with environmental concerns. Multilateral trade agreements and ongoing negotiation seek to ensure that free trade does not also lead to loss of biodiversity, environmental degradation or the accumulation of dangerous goods. The World Trade Organization (WTO) encourages businesses to act within the environmental laws of each country and the General Agreement on Trade and Tariffs (GATT) allows for exceptions to free trade if countries are concerned about environmental goals, safety or public health.

Understanding the pressures on health and the environment

The influences, or driving forces, outlined in this chapter provide the conditions that can avert or increase environmental health threats. Very often, more than one driving force is associated with a particular issue and dealing with the problems or opportunities they create can be very complex. How governments legislate and create programmes to deal with these driving forces is not only important but crucial in mitigating environmental health threats. It is not enough to understand how a factory might be polluting a community and the resultant risk to the population; the driving forces behind the threat must be taken into account. For instance, it is important to fully understand the structure of the population; the socio-economic status of the community; the technology needed to deal with the pollutant and the economic and political situation.

Hazards and risks in the environment

Now that you have a basic understanding of the interaction between environment and health, you can begin to examine specific risks and hazards posed by the environment to human health. This is necessary in order to protect human health and the environment. A hazard is defined as 'a factor or exposure that may adversely affect health' (Last 1995). This is basically a source of danger; it is a qualitative term used to express the potential of an environmental agent to harm particular individuals if the exposure is above a certain level. An example of a hazard might be pesticide 'X' sprayed on apples.

A risk is defined as 'the probability that an event will occur, e.g. that an individual will become ill or die within a stated period of time or age; the probability of a (generally) unfavourable outcome' (Last 1995). In other words, a risk is the quantitative probability that a health effect will occur after an individual has been exposed to a specified amount of hazard. An example of a risk is the chance of suffering cancer of the stomach after eating two apples a day for life (the exposure) which have been sprayed with pesticide 'X' (the hazard).

 Activity 3.3

There are many types of environmental health hazard; these may vary according to a country's or an area's state of development. List some environmental health hazards under two headings – traditional and modern. Traditional hazards are those that people have been exposed to in the agricultural and early industrial stages of development, while modern hazards mostly belong to the twentieth or twenty-first century and are associated with high population density and technological innovation.

Feedback

Table 3.4 illustrates some of the hazards you might have considered. Traditional hazards have been linked with lack of development, while modern hazards are associated with unsustainable development – in other words, development that lacks adequate mechanisms to protect human health or the environment.

Table 3.4 Examples of traditional and modern health hazards

Traditional hazards	Modern hazards
lack of access to safe drinking water	water pollution from populated areas or intensive agriculture
inadequate or poor quality housing and shelter	
inadequate basic sanitation (household and community)	urban air pollution from motor cars, coal power stations and industry; traffic accidents
food contamination with pathogens, dietary deficiency	food contamination with pesticides; poor diet leading to obesity
indoor air pollution from cooking and heating using biomass fuel (wood, animal dung and crop residues)	tobacco smoke
disease vectors, mainly insects and rodents	emerging and re-emerging infectious disease hazards *Continued*

Table 3.4 *Continued*

Traditional hazards	Modern hazards
inadequate solid waste disposal	solid and hazardous waste accumulation
occupational injury hazards in agriculture and cottage industries	chemical and radiation hazards following introduction of industrial and agricultural technologies
natural disasters, including floods, droughts and earthquakes	deforestation, land degradation and other major ecological changes at local and regional levels
	climate change, ozone depletion in the stratosphere and trans-boundary pollution

The risk transition

Risk transition is the process by which societies change exposure from traditional to modern hazards and is associated with economic development. This can be a problem if the transition is not well managed as there can be an overlap of traditional and modern hazards, leading to an extra health burden on society. The following extract from the WHO (1997) explains further.

 ## The environmental health risk transition

'Traditional' environmental health risks relating to unsafe food and drinking water; inadequate sanitation; infections from animals and vectors, and poor housing have a major influence on health when countries are at early stages of development. Industrial development introduces 'modern' environmental health risks relating to air pollution; chemical exposures and traffic accidents. The term 'risk transition' is used to describe the reduction in 'traditional risks' and increase in 'modern risks' that take place as economic development progresses. However, when environmental health risks are poorly managed, the 'traditional risks' are not eliminated in all parts of society and remain important health threats among the poor and disadvantaged, while the 'modern risks' continue unabated. But if environmental health risks are well managed, the 'traditional risks' can be eliminated almost completely and 'modern risk' reduced through effective prevention programmes.

Favourable completion of the environmental health risk transition can be threatened by the emergence of new infectious diseases; the occurrence of old disease in geographic areas where they had not previously appeared, and the resurgence of old diseases that had once appeared to be under control. In some countries, the revival of traditional health risks of this type is the result of poorly- managed and inequitable development. Associated factors are wide-ranging and include destruction of pristine areas; land use changes; resource extraction and agricultural exploitation; introduction of new agricultural and animal husbandry methods; increasing spread of drug-resistant pathogens and pesticide resistance in vectors; increased mobility of people and foodstuffs and changing lifestyles and eating habits.

Managing the risk transition also involves preventing or minimising modern environmental health risks. These can arise from the very modernisation activities that help lower traditional risks.

Activity 3.4

The authors touch on methods required to ensure that new risks are kept to a minimum and traditional risks are eliminated. What are these?

Feedback

In order to complete the health risk transition favourably, the authors emphasize the need for 'equitable development'; good management and effective prevention programmes. These require committed leadership; substantial long-term investment of resources; coordination across all relevant sectors including health, transport, housing, environment, etc.; long-term planning, monitoring and target setting, possibly including penalties for defaulters. These measures can prevent the advance of new diseases, the resurgence of old ones, the destruction of land, the introduction of new drug-resistant pathogens and pollution and lifestyle changes likely to promote ill health.

Summary

You will have seen the importance of human driving forces – such as population, poverty, technology and economics – in alleviating or exacerbating the effect of the environment on health. There are many types of environmental hazard, from such traditional dangers as lack of access to safe water to the modern perils of noxious waste accumulation. How societies move from traditional to modern hazards is known as the 'risk transition' and is of growing significance in the developing world, where governments and individuals often have to cope with both types of hazard simultaneously.

References

EIA (2005) http://www.eia.doe.gov/emeu/cabs/archives/china/part1.html. Accessed 14 February 2005.

Intermediate Technology Development Group: http://itdg.org/?id=new_technologies_case_ studies. Accessed September 2004.

Kuby M, Harner J and Gober P (1998) *Human Geography in Action*. New York: John Wiley & Sons Ltd.

Last A (1995) *A Dictionary of Epidemiology* (3rd edn). New York: Oxford University Press.

Sarre P and Blunden J (1996) *Environment, Population and Development*. Buckingham: Open University Press.

UN (2001) *Road Map towards the Implementation of the United Nations Millennium Declaration: Report of the Secretary-General*. New York: United Nations.

UN (2004) *Implementation of the United Nations Millennium Declaration: Report of the Secretary-General*. New York: United Nations.

UNDP (2003) *Human Development Report 2003: Millennium Development Goals: A Compact among Nations to End Human Poverty*. New York: Oxford University Press. Available at: http://www.undp.org/hdr2003/

UNFPA (2004) *State of the World Population Report*. New York: UN.
WHO (1996) *World Health Report: Fighting Disease, Fostering Development*. Geneva: WHO.
WHO (1997) *Environment, Health and Sustainable Development*. Geneva: WHO.

Further reading

Millennium Development Goals: http://www.undp.org/mdg/
Population issues UN Population Fund: http://www.unfpa.org/
Science and Environment Health Network (NGO, useful information on the precautionary
    principle): http://www.sehn.org/
Smith KR (1997) Development, health, and the environmental risk transition, in Shahi G,
    Levy BS, Binger A, Kjellstrom T and Lawrence R (eds) *International Perspectives in
    Environment, Development, and Health*. New York: Springer, 51–62.
UN human development reports: http://hdr.undp.org/

SECTION 2

Environmental quality

4 Environmental quality and human activity

Overview

Human activity impacts upon the quality of the environment. In this chapter and the two that follow you will look at how different human activities such as industry, transport, energy and waste disposal can affect the environment and human health. Exposure to different sources of pollution may occur simultaneously or in isolation, and have a varying degree of impact upon human health. Sources of pollution are often complex, the same pollutant resulting from transport, energy production and industry. Some primary pollutants are converted into secondary pollutants in the environment and making changes to improve one area of pollution production may affect levels of pollution produced elsewhere.

Learning objectives

By the end of this chapter, you will be better able to:

- **describe the different ways that human activity affects the environment**
- **give examples of the different influences that industry has on both health and the environment**
- **describe the positive and negative effects of transport on the environment**

Key term

Biodiversity Variability among living organisms including the variability within and between species and within and between ecosystems.

Environmental quality and health

Maintaining and recycling resources obtained from the air, soil, water and the ecosystem are essential for the supply of safe food, drinking (potable) water and shelter. As the population grows, increasing demands are placed on the environment from the 'driving forces' of human societies (see Chapter 3). Air pollution, deforestation, land degradation, poor water quality and loss of biodiversity all become significant environmental threats. Through industrial exploitation of the environment for the benefit of humankind, waste has been created which cannot re-enter the natural cycle or be usefully recycled.

In other words, human activities such as transport, energy use, industry and agriculture put significant pressure on the environment. Air, water and food are the principal vectors by which the harmful results of these activities affect humans. This chapter introduces the some of the issues relating to environmental quality. You will read about these issues in more detail in later chapters; air pollution (Chapters 8 and 9); water pollution (Chapter 7); waste production (Chapter 6); energy production (Chapter 5); climate change and global issues (Chapters 10 and 14).

Environmental exposures and health

Contamination of water, air and soil by pollution can have an adverse effect upon human health. While we tend to concentrate on the health effects of single routes of exposure such as air pollution or waste disposal, in reality, we are exposed to a cumulative number of environmental hazards, all of which impact upon our health. It is therefore a challenge to recognize the variety of exposures and act to mitigate these. Exposure to indoor air pollution, particularly in developing countries, has a significant adverse impact on health; however, there are other hazards in the domestic environment, such as contaminated water, poor waste disposal and over-/under-insulation, leading to houses that are too cold or too hot. It is important to consider the effect of all of these exposures on health, not just one in isolation.

Activity 4.1

You have read about the wide range of environmental hazards that humans are exposed to. Some diseases are associated with a range of environmental exposures – acute respiratory disease, for instance, is associated with poor housing, overcrowding and indoor air pollution. This means that complex solutions are required to reduce the burden of environmental-related diseases; both indoor and outdoor air pollution need to be targeted to have an impact upon acute respiratory disease.

Table 4.1 details specific health conditions and specific environmental exposures – tick those boxes where you believe an association exists between exposure risk and health condition.

Table 4.1 Potential associations between exposure and health

Health conditions	Polluted air	Excreta and household waste	Polluted water or deficiencies in water management	Polluted food	Unhealthy housing	Global environment change
Acute respiratory disease	✓				✓	
Diarrhoeal disease						
Other infections						
Malaria, other vector-borne diseases						
Injuries and poisonings						
Mental health conditions						
Cardiopulmonary diseases						
Cancer						
Chronic respiratory diseases						

Source: Adapted from WHO (1997)

 Feedback

Human health is clearly associated with exposure to a variety of pollutants which need to be taken into account when developing health policies. For example, concentrating resources on tackling unhealthy housing will be associated with a positive impact on a range of health conditions including respiratory disease, injuries, cardiovascular disease, cancer and mental illness. If diarrhoea is to be tackled effectively, then policies relating to polluted food and water *as well as* waste disposal needs to be developed.

Table 4.2 Potential associations between exposure and health

Health conditions	Polluted air	Excreta and household waste	Polluted water or deficiencies in water management	Polluted food	Unhealthy housing	Global environment change
Acute respiratory disease	✓				✓	
Diarrhoeal disease		✓	✓	✓	✓	✓
Other infections		✓	✓	✓	✓	
Malaria, other vector-borne diseases		✓	✓		✓	✓
Injuries and poisonings	✓		✓	✓	✓	✓
Mental health conditions					✓	
Cardiopulmonary diseases	✓					✓
Cancer	✓			✓		✓
Chronic respiratory diseases	✓				✓	✓

Source: Adapted from WHO (1997)

Industry

Industrialization is essential for economic development, however, if it is uncontrolled, it can be a major source of pollution. Developed countries are still responsible for 75 per cent of global industrial production, although this is changing as increasing areas of the world are undergoing rapid industrialization, particularly, for instance, in South-East Asia. Industry accounts for 32 per cent of the world's Gross Domestic Product (GDP) whereas agriculture accounts for only 4 per cent (and the service sector accounts for 64 per cent). Thus industry is vital to the economy of many countries. The nature of industry is changing; whereas it was once dominated by extraction and manufacturing, now, at least in developed countries, there is an increase in new technology-based industries such as computing, robotics, telecommunications, pharmaceuticals and medical equipment. Rapid development of new industrial and agricultural technology has meant that there are new challenges to the environment.

Activity 4.2

Make a list of the ways in which industry might have an impact on the environment and therefore on health.

⟳ **Feedback**

Industry impacts upon the environment and health in a number of positive and negative ways. Your list may contain some of the suggestions below.

Negative impacts of industry

- energy use and resource depletion
- water consumption, again depleting resources available for domestic use
- creation and disposal of solid and hazardous wastes
- air and water pollution

Positive impacts of industry

- job creation
- enhanced communications with rural or marginalized communities

The creation of pollution and waste related to industry is a consequence of routine discharges, but also as a result of accidental releases which may have serious environmental consequences. This last point is discussed more fully in Chapter 12.

As industry grows, so too will its impact upon the environment. There are likely to be increases in industrial pollution as well as an escalation of resources depletion. How the environment will be affected will depend on emerging industries as well as changes in technology.

Industrial resources and emissions

Industry relies very heavily on transport (the intake of raw materials and the later shipment of processed products, for example), and draws heavily on local or imported energy sources. As such, it is a major source of air and water, noise and other waste pollutants, some of them hazardous. The health of both the workforce and the general population is directly affected by industry, not only through daily discharges of waste into the environment, but also because of industrial accidents. The environmental and health impacts of energy use are discussed in more detail in Chapter 5.

Various industries have the potential for wide contamination of the environment, including the pollution of air, water and soil. For example, the coal mining industry can contribute significantly to air pollution through dust (from extraction, storage and transportation), burning slag heaps and the risk of fire and explosion. Both surface and ground water can be contaminated with mine water and the land is damaged by disturbance, erosion and subsidence as well as the placing of large slag heaps of material that cannot be used for other purposes. Other industries have similarly wide-reaching environmental effects, many of them more potentially damaging. Exactly how the industry will affect the environment depends mainly on the nature of the emissions and these include:

- product – the type and scale of production
- the manufacturing process

- raw materials – what is used and in what quantities, including the energy for transport to the plant and any involved in extraction
- use of natural resources during the manufacturing process, such as water and air
- use of energy – its source and quantity required
- size of manufacturing plant
- amount of toxic material stored at site
- quality and efficiency of abatement technology – if any.

Other important considerations are:

- natural environmental conditions – topography, rivers, soil type, wind, etc.
- location of human settlements (WHO 1997).

This list clearly shows that the environmental impact of industry is not only as a result of the manufacturing process, but also arises from the collection of raw materials, the production of energy, transport and final destination of the goods. A further important factor is also the impact of the disposal of the packaging waste and, eventually, the goods themselves.

With the Industrial Revolution in the UK (1760–1830) and later, in other parts of the developed world, came air pollution. Textbooks that cover the Industrial Revolution contain many images of huge factories, belching out smoke over the surrounding areas. Modern industry, although better controlled, is still responsible for a large quantity of emissions of sulphur dioxide, carbon monoxide, nitrogen oxides (NO_x), hydrocarbons and particulates. In addition to these, some specific industries have their own specific chemical emissions associated with them; you will read more on the effects of the main pollutants in Chapter 8.

Water pollution can occur at several stages in the industrial process. Water may be used as part of the manufacturing process before being discharged back into waterways or onto soil, for example, as a coolant during the process of electricity generation. Other waste products may be released into rivers, streams, lakes or seas. It is worth pointing out, however, that although water pollution may affect the quality of the water and the ecological balance in the environment, it may not damage human health directly.

Soil contamination can occur as a result of settling air pollution, precipitation or direct application. Dumping of waste can lead to water pollution if there is subsequent leaching or run-off into a water source. In Chapter 6, the fate of hazardous waste from a variety of industries is considered in more detail.

Activity 4.3

1 Significant pollution can be discharged by small-scale industries. What are the potential detriments and benefits of small-scale industry for both the environment and human health?

2 Note the direct effects of industry on the workers involved. Are they beneficial or damaging?

3 A further important feature of the relationship between industry and health is the occurrence of occupational accidents. These have the potential to significantly affect workers' health, particularly in areas with few or poor regulations for industrial and working practices. Figures 4.1 and 4.2 demonstrate workplace fatalities in

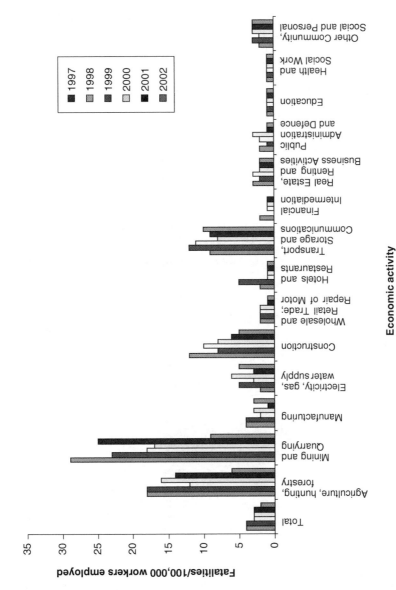

Figure 4.1 Fatal workplace injuries by occupational sector, Australia, 1997–2002

Source: ILO, LABORSTA Labour Statistics Database. Geneva

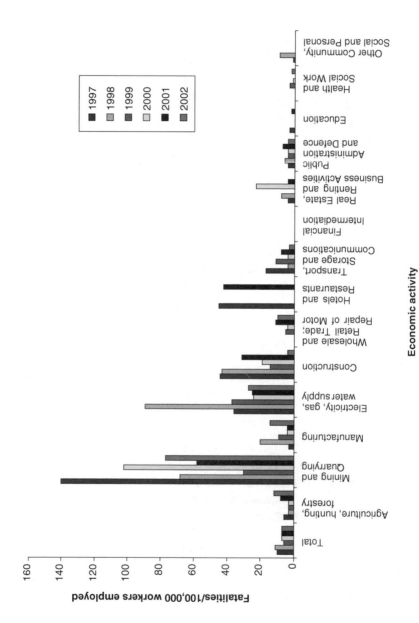

Figure 4.2 Fatal workplace injuries by occupational sector, Kyrgyzstan, 1997–2002

Source: ILO, LABORSTA Labour Statistics Database. Geneva

Australia, a high income country in the Pacific, and Kyrgyzstan, a country in transition that was previously part of the Soviet Union. Compare these graphs and note down the differences and similarities in the trends and overall rates in the two countries.

↻ Feedback

1 Small industry brings the environmental impact of waste disposal and air pollution directly to the local community, counteracting those potential benefits provided by employment of the local population. This has a greater impact in developing countries, where small-scale industry tends to dominate, contributing substantially to the local economy. Small-scale industries such as mining and metal smelting are very polluting. The proximity of these industries to human settlements can lead to serious environmental and health problems. These industries can be made more efficient and less polluting by the use of environmentally sustainable technologies, but unfortunately these technologies are often expensive or difficult to source. The regulation of small-scale industry is a problem for developing countries; the industry provides much needed income and employment for the local area as well as for the associated services such as shops, food outlets and transport and so regulators are often reluctant to intervene. Industry is essential for local development and prosperity and brings health benefits directly through work and a strong economy. Policy makers must strike a balance between economic progress and the environmental imperatives of sustainable development.

2 The most significant effect upon health by industry is employment – employed people have better health than unemployed people and are better able to afford good quality services, housing, food, and other goods for themselves and their families. However, working in some industries leads to exposure to pollution from air, water and solid waste which could be potentially harmful to health.

3 There are more than twice as many fatal accidents per 100 000 workers in Kyrgyzstan – 8 per 100 000 compared with 3.2 per 100 000 in Australia. Rates have fallen in both countries over the period covered.

Mining and quarrying are the major contributors to workplace fatalities in Kyrgyzstan. The reason isn't given but one can surmise that it could be due to the scale of the industry or to poor occupational health and safety regulations. Australia has very strict regulations to protect workers and members of the public.

The International Labour Organization (ILO) believes that there is under-reporting of accidents, particularly in the informal sector of an economy. A far greater number of non-fatal injuries are reported in Australia than in Kyrgyzstan. This may be because Australia bases its figures on compensation claims for injury so there is an incentive for the worker or employer to notify the accident. Compensation is more likely to be paid in a high income economy. In Kyrgyzstan the figures are based on the official labour inspectorate. It is possible that injuries are under-reported, so as not to draw attention to the poorly managed plant/industry and its working practices. It is also possible that managers report serious injuries but not *all* injuries. A further complication is a lack of standardization in data collection and reporting; as different countries collect data in different ways, it is difficult to make comparisons of occupational injury rates between them.

The impacts of rapid industrialization

Areas of rapid industrialization, such as the 'tiger' economies of the eastern Pacific, have experienced considerable environmental change, with consequent effects on public health. Industrial pollution rises very quickly in newly developing regions (Landon et al. 1998), and this brings about a number of 'knock-on' effects. These effects are due not only to the industry itself, but also to financial and employment growth and an increase in the provision of services. In Thailand, for example, as the gross domestic product doubled between 1975 and 1989, atmospheric pollution increased tenfold! With increasing wealth, there was more money available for people to progress from bicycles to scooters and from scooters to cars. Typically, in such circumstances, little thought and planning was directed towards mass transport systems, and private vehicle ownership becomes even more important as a mark of status. Urban planning becomes crucial to prevent large squatter and slum developments from forming and to provide essential services to the growing population. There is more detail on urbanization in Chapter 13.

Sustainable development and industry

Sustainable development of industry is seen as helping to protect not only the environment, but also the workers and communities around that industry. The question has been raised as to whether the economic and other pressures on industry are compatible with sustainable development. A large study on 'Greening Industry' by the World Bank (World Bank 1999), looked at how in the late 1990s, industrial pollution in low and middle income countries was decreasing through economic and regulatory policy reforms, but without threatening important economic growth. The regulatory models used in high income countries had failed, and new models were being created, involving new methods of pollution control, based on good economic principles. These initiatives are founded on market incentives that are placed alongside commitments to make environmental information publicly available. There is also back-up assistance provided, specifically targeted at improving environmental control by plant managers. This model allows for the sustainable development of industry and the participation of all relevant interest groups, with communities represented alongside the government regulators and the factory owners. Since the Greening Industry Study was published, those responsible for environmental regulation in various countries have adopted some of the regulatory tools. The public information disclosure programme was originally designed and launched in Indonesia and, as a result of its success, has also been adopted in the People's Republic of China, the Philippines, Thailand, Vietnam and India, either as pilot or nation-wide programmes. Even in areas where there have been no formal meetings between the researchers and regulators, there are some interesting initiatives being undertaken. For example, in Iran, industries identified as good environmental performers are publicly named and congratulated. The outcome of the 'Greening Industry' policy has been to demonstrate how countries can adapt their regulatory systems for industry to promote both sustainable development and economic growth. The next activity looks at how environmental management of small industries in India is rising to meet these challenges.

Activity 4.4

The extract below by D'Souza (2001) discusses the integration of environmental management in small industries in India. As you read the extract consider the following questions:

1 What are the main pressures (driving forces) on the environment in India?
2 What is a possible method for sustainable business practice?
3 Why should India adopt sustainable business practices?
4 What are the issues surrounding compliance and regulation?

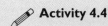 **Integrating environmental management in small industries of India**

The major environmental concerns in India today are poverty coupled with growing population and the side-effects of enhanced industrial activities. As long as poverty remains the main stumbling block, industrialization provides hope of significantly improving the standard of living . . . Removal of poverty and environmental protection are two sides of the same coin that is sustainable but policy makers, governments, politicians, and industrialists have challenged many of the underlying values and assumptions of sustainability . . .

. . . Where high population and economic growth demands resources (inputs) and discharges (outputs) in the form of pollutants, not many industries have arrived at suitable suggestions on sustainable measures, thus putting pressure on the environment . . . the problem of a growing population, rapid economic development in emerging economies, and political and social issues that exceed the mandate and the capabilities of any corporation. However, the suggestion that learning to balance ecological principles, economic growth, and social responsibility be priorities of businesses does eventually make more sense. Sustainable development challenges industry to produce high levels of output while using lower levels of inputs and generating less waste with a more effective use of raw materials in production that would eventually result in diminishing costs. This greener corporate image could then lead to an increased market share . . . the business logic for greening has been largely operational or technical, and bottom up pollution prevention programs have saved billions of dollars, but few have realised that environmental opportunities might actually become a major source of revenue growth . . . the concept of sustainable development should . . . be the core objective within the operations of small industries.

Small industries could also go one step further in addressing a sustainable vision i.e. a trade-off between economic growth, profitability, and sustainable environment . . . One such measure is Johannson's . . . trisect of sustainable business. It is founded on the concept of balancing ecology, economic, and social factors that are included in the industry's value system, and included in the business planning or design phase resulting in profits through ecologically sound products, processes, or services. In a complex relationship between population, economy, industry, and ecology, managing the environmental responsibility is a prime issue in India . . . regulation, compliance, and environmental laws will take care of themselves if managers adopt a sustainable vision or green objectives for industries. Much of the literature seeks to establish that there is an acute need for regulatory and legal measures. However, pressure for sustainable vision in these small industries lies within themselves. They must realize the importance of environmental management and quality and that it could be highly effective if it is administered by the small units themselves.

Feedback

I In India the population is still growing and the environment is affected as a result of poverty and a rapid growth in industry, much of it small-scale.

2 Three factors – the ecology, economic growth, and social responsibility – need to be part of the industry's value system, and included in business planning and design.

3 Industry provides economic growth and increases employment levels. However, industry will inevitably produce discharges and wastes that are capable of polluting and increasing pressure upon the environment. Sustainable business practices need to allow for both industrial growth *and* economic growth.

4 It is suggested that if managers are environmentally aware and adopt sustainable or green objectives for industries, regulation, compliance, and environmental laws will take care of themselves.

Transport

The quality of the environment is heavily influenced by transport systems, particularly in urban areas. The road and rail network allows goods and people to migrate and can bring communities and services together. However, it may also serve as an obstacle, separating local communities and creating the potential for accidents, especially for children at play. Planning for the environmental impact of transport systems is important, for instance, the need to segregate housing from major transport links, as well as taking account of engine emissions which are major contributors to air pollution. The rest of this chapter is primarily concerned with road transport. There are of course many other forms of transport which are not investigated in detail in this chapter, for example, animal, rail, air and water-based forms of transport. All these contribute to the economy and have different environmental impacts.

What are the environmental impacts arising from the production of road vehicles and their use? Motor vehicle manufacture consumes large amounts of energy and resources, generating considerable waste, including the disposal of old, redundant vehicles. After manufacture, driving causes significant air pollution (nitrogen oxides (NO_x), carbon monoxide and volatile organic compounds); many of these, together with the water vapour produced, are greenhouse gases. Another environmental impact comes from the construction and maintenance of road systems, with consequences for air pollution, water pollution, habitat destruction and stream sedimentation.

 Activity 4.5

List the health-promoting and damaging effects of road transport on health.

Feedback

> Table 4.3 has some ideas; you may have included others. You may have noticed that
> this does not allow for the variety in scale of health-promoting and health-damaging
> factors associated with different forms of road transport. For example, one can note
> that driving a bus is polluting, whereas travelling by bicycle is more environmentally
> friendly. However, a bus can transport more people than other forms of road transport
> and cyclists are at greater risk of road traffic accidents compared to bus passengers.

> **Table 4.3** Health-promoting and health-damaging effects related to road transport
>
> | Health effect | Results |
> | --- | --- |
> | Promoting | enables access to: employment; education; shops; recreation; social support networks; health services; countryside
provides recreation and exercise |
> | Damaging | accidents
pollution: carbon monoxide; nitrogen oxides; hydrocarbons; ozone; carbon dioxide; lead; benzene
noise and vibration
stress and anxiety
loss of land and planning blight
severance of communities by roads |
>
> Source: Adapted from Whitelegg (1993)

Transport and air pollution

Transport has a significant effect on air quality; it is responsible for over 50 per
cent of nitrogen dioxide, carbon monoxide and hydrocarbon pollution in Europe
(Whitelegg 1993). As countries develop, there is increased reliance on transport – to
move people, food, raw and processed goods and waste. Improving economies, and
rising income levels, have led to an increase in the demand for personal transport
and a resultant huge increase in motor vehicle ownership. In 1965 there were 60
vehicles per 1,000 people on the roads, by 1996 there were more than 140 vehicles
per 1,000 people world-wide (AAMA 1996). In the People's Republic of China the
vehicle fleet grew 700 per cent in this period and is still expanding rapidly. To
provide the energy for this expansion of transport there has been a large increase
in the consumption of fossil fuels. These are responsible for a large proportion of
gaseous pollutants. Diesel engines that are poorly maintained are responsible for
most of the fine particulate emissions. The potentially serious health implications
of air pollution related to transport are discussed in Chapter 8. The increased use of
fossil fuels contributes to climate change and finding ways to make transport more
sustainable will make an important contribution to climate change mitigation.

Another environmental burden from road transport has been the significant levels
of lead pollution associated with the use of leaded gasoline. Lead was added to
gasoline to enhance engine performance and has been shown to be associated with
a reduction in children's intelligence rating and their mental development

(Fewtrell et al. 2004). Alternative additives have been found for petrol and in many parts of the world, lead additives to fuels are now banned.

The pollutants emitted by gasoline-powered vehicles and the particulates given off by diesel have a disproportionate and growing effect on the environment, particularly because they are released at ground level, influencing carbon monoxide and ozone levels in the cities.

Transport and accidents

Road traffic accidents are the most important cause of non-accidental injury world-wide and so are a major health problem. These accidents were ranked as the ninth most important reason for loss of Disability Adjusted Life Years (DALYs) in 1990 (Murray and Lopez 1997). As with the air pollution associated with transport, there is a direct correlation between increasing levels of accidents and a rapid increase in motor vehicle ownership; this decreases when the infrastructure (roads, safety promotion and better vehicles) improves. Low and middle income countries are therefore the most vulnerable to the effects of motor vehicle accidents, despite having far fewer vehicles on the road per head of population, because their infrastructure is least likely to be able to ameliorate the effects of motor vehicle ownership.

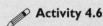

Activity 4.6

How do you get to work, to the shops, or visit friends and relatives? What is the average distance of your journey? If you use motorized transport, is there an alternative? What might be the benefits to the environment and to your health were you to begin cycling?

Feedback

If those who live within 1 or 2 kilometres of any destination walked or cycled instead of using a car, bus or motorcycle to get there, this would improve both personal fitness and the local environment. The use of a bus or train rather than individual motorized vehicles for longer journeys would also lessen any impact on the environment, although in some circumstances such as in very rural areas, this is not possible due to lack of public transport provision.

Potential benefits of walking or cycling are:

• time saving – no problems in parking or having to negotiate traffic jams
• exercise – important for cardiovascular fitness and helping to prevent obesity
• no addition to air pollution
• reclamation of urban space – smaller roads and fewer parking spaces required
• fewer cars and motorcycles produced – less industrial pollution and use of resources (although this would be accompanied by some economic dislocation)

Measures such as these could enable the principles of sustainable development to be met. You could conduct a similar exercise on the potential benefits of large food retailers to reduce transportation costs by selling locally-sourced produce instead of imported goods. Such alternatives need to be considered if changes in policy are to be made for the sake of improving the environment.

Summary

Industrial exposures affect human health at the individual and population level. There are, however, successful models of sustainable industrial development that support economic growth and allow countries to develop. Transport affects the quality of the environment and health, particularly in urban areas. Improving economies and rising incomes have led to an increased reliance on road transport that is required to move people, food, raw and processed goods. Moreover, we have seen a huge rise in motor vehicle ownership world-wide. Road transport is a major contributor to urban air pollution; as the numbers of vehicles in the road increase, countries will need to consider how to deal with the environmental and health impacts from pollution, accidents, road building and disposal of vehicles.

References

AAMA (American Automobile Manufacturers Association) (1996) *Motor Vehicle Fact and Figures 1996*. Washington, DC: AAMA.

CIA (2001) *The World Factbook 2002*. http://www.cia.gov/cia/publications/factbook/

D'Souza CM (2001) Integrating environmental management in small industries of India. *Electronic Green Journal* 14, Spring.

Fewtrell LJ, Pruss-Ustun A, Landrigan P and Ayuso-Mateos JL (2004) Estimating the global burden of disease of mild mental retardation and cardiovascular diseases from environmental lead exposure. *Environmental Research* 94(2): 120–33.

ILO, LABORSTA, Labour Statistics Database. Geneva. Extracted 10 September 2004.

Landon M, McVey D, Wilkinson P and Fletcher T (1998) International comparisons of the key factors affecting health: an analysis of the international databases on health, in *Key Players for a New Era: Leading Health Promotion into 21st Century*. WHO conference proceedings. Geneva: WHO.

Murray C and Lopez A (1997) Mortality by cause for the eight regions of the world: Global Burden of Disease Study. *Lancet* 349: 1269–76.

Whitelegg J (1993) *Transport for a Sustainable Future: The Case for Europe*. Chichester: John Wiley and Sons Ltd.

WHO (1997) *Environment, Health and Sustainable Development*. Geneva: WHO.

World Bank (1999) *Greening Industry: New Roles for Communities, Markets and Governments*. Washington, DC: World Bank.

Further reading

Sustainable transport: www.sustrans.org.uk/

United Nations: Sustainability and industry: www.un.org/esa/sustdev/sdissues/industry/industry.htm

World Resources Institute: http://earthtrends.wri.org/

Energy use and sustainable development

Overview

Energy is essential for human activity. As populations increase and there is greater prosperity, the demand for energy also increases. Currently the world is dependent on oil for most of its energy. However, the limited supply of oil and other sources of energy will become an increasingly important problem. The production and consumption of energy can contribute to both indoor and outdoor pollution and therefore can negatively impact on the quality of the environment. There are positive and negative health impacts of the use of energy and these must be balanced. This chapter looks in detail at the direct and indirect effects of different energy sources and the role that energy production can play in sustainable development.

Learning objectives

By the end of this chapter, you will be better able to:

- **describe the direct and indirect health effects associated with different energy sources**
- **give examples of the different methods of energy production and their effects on human health**
- **understand the principles that should be used when considering sustainable energy development**

Key terms

Radionuclide Nuclide (an atom that exists for a measurable length of time) that decays, producing radioactive particles or rays. Radionuclides may be natural or synthetically produced.

Relative risk Estimate of the magnitude of an association between exposure and disease and indicates the likelihood of developing the disease in those exposed relative to those unexposed.

Sievert (Sv) A unit equivalent dose of radiation which relates the absorbed dose in human tissue to the effective biological damage of the radiation. A milisievert (mSv) is one thousandth of a sievert.

Energy – production and consumption

Access to energy sources for personal use is considered to be a basic human need. Energy consumption varies widely throughout the world and is related to social development. As societies develop economically, their energy requirements change. An agriculture-based society will use five times more energy than a hunter–gatherer society, and a technological society at least fifty times more. Clearly, as economies around the world have developed from agriculture-based to technology-based, world rates of energy consumption have increased.

 Activity 5.1

Think about the different types of energy you use in your everyday life and note down the reasons you use it, and if known, its source.

 Feedback

There are many different sources of energy requirements, and you will almost certainly have noted some of these:

- basic human needs – heating, lighting, cooking (using electricity, oil, biomass fuel)
- agriculture – irrigation, mechanization (using wind, oil, electricity, water)
- urbanization – basic services for city life (using oil, electricity, coal)
- transport (using oil, physical (cycling), electricity)
- industry (using electricity, oil, coal, wind, water)

In all these cases, the electricity used has itself to be produced from oil, coal, gas, hydroelectric methods or nuclear power.

Positive and negative impacts of energy consumption on health

The production and consumption of energy have significant positive and negative impacts on the environment and on health. The provision of heat in homes can be seen as positive, along with the provision of energy for cooking food, providing power for water supply, health services, and educational facilities, and so on. Energy consumption increases with economic advancement and this is linked to improvements in health and, through work, access to services and social activities. There are, however, significant negative health effects to consider, and these may be distributed unequally among different groups. The largest source of outdoor air pollution stems from the use of fossil fuels in power plants, industry and transport. Indoor pollution from the use of biomass fuels (such as wood, animal dung and crop residues) is a significant health threat to hundreds of millions of people. The health impacts of these outdoor and indoor pollutants are considered in more detail in Chapters 8 and 9 respectively.

Other forms of energy production such as solar power, wind power, tidal/ wave power, hydroelectricity and nuclear energy are less common in low and middle income countries and so arguably have a smaller environmental impact (Moeller 1997). However, there are concerns, particularly over the building of big dams for hydroelectricity production, about the environmental and social cost of these development projects. Nuclear power only supplies a relatively small number of people with power and although it is energy-producing it has, on the whole, resulted in only minor environmental impact; it causes public concern because of the possibility of a further accident such as the one at Chernobyl in the Ukraine in 1986. There are also huge costs and uncertain risks associated with the decommissioning of nuclear plants and the safe disposal of radioactive waste.

The negative impacts of energy production and consumption are not only local, but also carry regional and global climate change consequences which are of concern for the achievement of sustainable development.

Energy resources

There are a number of resources available for use in the production of energy (Table 5.1). The world's energy production is dominated by non-renewable sources of energy (Table 5.1), mostly oil. By comparison, renewable energy sources have little impact on world energy consumption (with the exception of biomass fuels). Renewable energy sources may prove important in achieving sustainable development in the future.

Table 5.1 World energy consumption of non-renewable and renewable sources of energy in 2002

Non-renewable (%)	Renewable (%)
solid fuels 23 (coal, lignite, peat)	biomass fuels 11 (wood, crop residues and dung)
oil (36)	hydroelectricity (dams) 2
natural gas 21	geothermal heat 0.4
	wind, solar, tides/waves, less than 0.1
uranium – nuclear power 7	

Source: IEA/OECD (2004)

Nearly two-thirds of the world-wide consumption of energy occurs in high income countries, despite their having only 22 per cent of the world population. The per capita energy consumption in low and middle income countries is only 18 per cent that of the high income countries. As low and middle income countries industrialize and motorized transport increases, the per capita consumption has to increase; the global challenge will be to provide enough energy for all who require it, while minimizing the effect on the environment. Table 5.2 shows that energy use (as measured against gross domestic product (GDP)) has fallen in most country groups since 1990, but has risen in Western Asia and the Commonwealth of Independent States.

Table 5.2 Energy use (consumption of kg oil equivalent) per $1,000 gross domestic product (GDP (PPP) (Indicator 27 of the Millennium Goals)

	1990	2001
Latin America and the Caribbean	187	177
Northern Africa	202	196
Sub-Saharan Africa	400	406
Eastern Asia	294	216
Southern Asia	326	256
South-Eastern Asia	223	237
Western Asia	268	327
Oceania	...	...
Commonwealth of Independent States	613	644
Transition countries in Europe(a)	527	484
High-income countries(b)	233	214

(a) Including transition countries in Europe classified by the World Bank as low or middle income economies.
(b) As defined by the World Bank.

Source: UN (2004)

Sustainable development and energy use

Sustainable development is a central tenet of the achievement of the Millennium Goals, as discussed in Chapter 3. Goal number seven relates specifically to sustainable development and three of the indicators relate to energy use and are outlined below:

- energy use (kg oil equivalent) per $1 (US) GDP (PPP)
- carbon dioxide emissions per capita and consumption of ozone-depleting chlorofluorocarbons (CFCs)
- proportion of population using solid fuels.

If these indicators can be reduced in line with the targets set out in the Millennium Declaration, there will be a significant benefit to human health.

The rest of this chapter covers the positive and negative health and environmental impacts of energy use. As you read, relate the issues back to the Millennium Goal targets to understand the potential benefits from reaching these targets. The significance of reducing carbon dioxide emissions is covered in Chapter 10.

Development and energy production

There have been huge increases in commercial energy production since the Industrial Revolution, and this is increasing at an even greater pace as more countries take advantage of economic growth and access to mechanized and other technologies. The increase in commercial energy production is due to a number of factors (Gupta and Asher 1998), primarily:

- increasing population, driving demand for energy
- increase in energy-intensive consumption
- rapid industrialization
- growth of mechanized transport.

Most energy consumption and production takes place in high income countries but, as energy production changes as a result of the factors listed above, these figures will increase and the role of the low and middle income nations in energy consumption and production will start to predominate.

Energy use and environmental degradation

The rapid increase in the production and consumption of energy world-wide is associated with an increase in environmental degradation through a number of mechanisms, including:

- deforestation and habitat destruction associated with wood collection for use as fuel
- air pollution (indoor and outdoor) through the burning of solid fuel and petroleum derivatives; also pollution of soil and water
- environmental problems associated with large-scale hydroelectric dam projects
- release of radioactive matter (arguably the most dangerous).

Power generation

The generation of power creates a variety of pollutants, depending on the method of production. Table 5.3 outlines these in more detail for the three main sources of energy: fossil fuels, nuclear and hydroelectricity. Note the wide range of pollutants associated with fossil fuels in particular. The following section considers each of these sources of energy in more detail.

Hydroelectricity

Hydroelectric power is generated by building a dam across a stream or river and creating a reservoir of water. The water, with its potential energy, is then forced to flow through pipes that spin turbines and generate electricity.

Table 5.3 Major pollutants of power generation

Type of plant	Air	Water	Soil
Fossil fuel	Carbon monoxide (CO) Carbon dioxide (CO_2) Nitrogen dioxide (NO_2) Particulates Sulphur dioxide (SO_2) Volatile compounds organic	Acids and bases Hydrocarbons Metals Oil PCBs* Organic solvents	Acids/ bases Ash Hydrocarbons Metals Oil PCBs* Organic solvents
Nuclear	Radioactive emissions		
Hydro-electric		Chiefly leachates from to water behind dams All plants may result in discharge of warm water	

Note: *polychlorinated biphenyls
Source: Adapted from Pittman (1998)

Activity 5.2

Read the extract below from the International Rivers Network (2005) and the Chinese Embassy (2005) and consider what are the environmental and health impacts likely from the generation of hydroelectric power. Consider the building of the dam as well as the generation of power.

 Three Gorges Dam project

The Three Gorges Dam on the Yangtze river in China is the largest hydroelectric dam project in the world. The dam is designed to stretch over two kilometres across and tower 200 metres above the world's third longest river, its reservoir will stretch nearly 700 kilometres upstream. Construction began in 1994, is scheduled to take 20 years and has spiralling costs. The Chinese Government is very supportive of the project and sees it as a symbol of China's development and 'superior organizing.' The Chinese are proud of the scale of construction and the investment in new industries in the area. The scheme is designed to lessen flooding and make navigation of the river easier as well as to replace coal burning for electricity production.

Many environmentalists consider the Three Gorges Dam as the world's most environmentally and socially destructive infrastructure project:

• 1.8 million people will lose their homes and livelihoods
• fertile agricultural lands would be destroyed
• important cultural and historical sites will be flooded and lost
• loss of many species
• untreated industrial and domestic wastewater will no longer be flushed downstream
• flooding problems will continue, the reservoir will fill with silt within 50 years, impeding power production and navigation and increasing the chance of a catastrophic collapse

Much of the current emphasis is on human rights violations and inadequate settlement provisions and there has been controversy concerning funding and corruption around the construction process. This has led campaigners to question whether the project should continue.

 Feedback

The human health impacts from dam construction are mainly associated with construction and loss of land and property (Table 5.4). Displacement of populations and loss of agricultural and other land is a serious concern, particularly in high-density developing countries. There has been a lot of controversy surrounding the Three Gorges Dam project in China for this reason; having to relocate and find new employment or business creates economic and psychological stress. Once the dam is built and the hydroelectric power is being generated, the main impacts upon human health in many countries come from water-related diseases such as malaria and schistomastis. There is very little environmental pollution from hydroelectric power once the dam has been built, and the reservoir filled.

Table 5.4 Environmental and health impacts from hydroelectricity production

Environmental impact	Human health impact
catastrophic floods due to dam failure	loss of life and injury
changed environmental conditions for waterborne diseases	increase in waterborne diseases
decreased natural fertilization of downstream agricultural land	reduced crop planting, could lead to reduced food supply
loss of agricultural and other land	reduced ability to grow crops or graze animals for food
destroys wildlife habitats	
decreases fish harvests below the dam, prevents fish from migrating upstream to spawn (breed)	reduced fishing potential – although fish can be encouraged to breed in the artificial reservoirs
contamination of fish and aquatic ecology as well as greenhouse gas emissions (CO_2 and methane) due to decay of flooded forest and vegetation biomass	reduced harvest, also indirect effect on health through global climate change
occupational accidents during construction of dams and reservoirs	death and injury
dust and airborne pollution from construction and road building (respiratory symptoms)	respiratory symptoms
increased transport of building materials (air pollution and accidents)	respiratory symptoms, injury
populations displaced by building dams and filling reservoirs additional environmental impacts as they relocate to another area	psychological and economic stress

Fossil fuels

The burning of fossil fuels for power generation is one of the major sources of outdoor air pollution. Refer back to Table 5.3 and note the range of pollutants that are emitted – soil and water are affected as well as air. Not all fossil fuels generate the same amount of pollution; natural gas is the cleanest, whereas most oil will burn more cleanly than coal. The pollution generated by each type of fuel depends on the amount of non-combustible material contained, and each type of fuel is graded, depending on how polluting it is. For instance, so-called 'brown coal' is highly polluting as it contains more unfossilized material than other types of coal. Brown coal is also linked with the production of acidification, which is dealt with in more detail in Chapter 11. However, the ultimate concentrations of pollutants released from the fuel depend on a variety of factors; the type of burning technology used; any pollution control methods in place; the design and height of chimneys and geographical and meteorological conditions. As a result, pollution need not be airborne; it can remain in a solid form and be disposed of in another way.

Nuclear power

The primary health concern from nuclear power is the release of radioactive material. These effects on health from materials with a long half-life (they will remain in the environment for thousands of years), take place via inhalation from the air, external exposure from ground contamination and ingestion of foods from contaminated ground (Ahern et al. 2004). Exposure can lead to cancer and the potential for mutation, resulting in hereditary effects.

The fuel for nuclear power comes from uranium mining, although fuel is increasingly being generated in fast breeder reactors. Workers can inhale dust and be affected by the release of radionuclides. There have been a number of studies that show an excess of lung cancer in uranium mine workers. These effects can take many years to develop and only now are we experiencing health problems arising from mining done in the 1940s and 1950s. As more evidence has come to light, safety procedures have been improved to reduce worker exposure to radon decay products. It is also becoming clear that a low-level dose over a longer time may be more detrimental than a short-term high-level dose (Ahern et al. 2004).

Fewer studies have been carried out on populations living near uranium mines. Soil samples taken from surrounding areas show higher levels of contamination than in control areas and residents may be exposed to low levels of radioactive contamination for many years, leading to increased health risks.

There is also potential exposure to radionuclides from the waste materials from mining, processing, and power generation. High-level waste material is destined for deep geological burial, although this is controversial, due to public concerns about safety. A study of 90,000 USA and European power station employees found that exposure to low-level doses of radiation over a long period of time increased their risk of developing leukaemia.

Other concerns associated with nuclear power are that there could be the detonation of a nuclear weapon; the dispersal of radionuclides in conventional weapons; the crash of a vehicle transporting nuclear material; or another incident similar to the accident at the Chernobyl nuclear power plant in the former USSR (now Ukraine) in 1986. When an explosion blew the roof off one of the reactors, radioactive material was spread over a wide area up to 2,000 km from the plant. There were a number of direct health impacts observed as a result of the ionizing radiation from the release of radionuclides as well as the result of stress and relocation.

The three main groups affected were: workers at the plant and clean-up workers (especially those active in the first two years of decontamination); resident populations living in areas of high deposition of radionuclides; and the populations who were moved quickly to avoid radiation exposure. As a direct result of the explosion, there were two deaths and 134 reported cases of radiation sickness, 28 of whom died as a result of exposure to radiation in the first three months. There has been much research activity since the explosion to measure whether cancer rates have increased, and to estimate the health of both the residents in the immediate vicinity as well as those who were relocated to other areas. Marked increases in the incidence of thyroid cancer have occurred over a relatively limited period of observation in all areas of the Republic of Belarus and Ukraine, among all age categories. The greatest increases have occurred among children, suggesting that a high prevalence of pre-existing iodine deficiency, combined with unique suscepti-bility among younger people, might have contributed to potential carcinogenic exposures to the thyroid. Children born after the accident have a much lower prevalence of cancers and this cohort effect will wear out. There were no excess leukaemia or other cancers found, contrary to what might have been expected from the experience of the nuclear bomb exposures. The effects on crops and animals at greater distances from the plant are still under study.

Nuclear fuel cycle

All energy sources have a fuel cycle, beginning at the stage of mining or extraction and ending with their disposal. There are impacts on the environment and

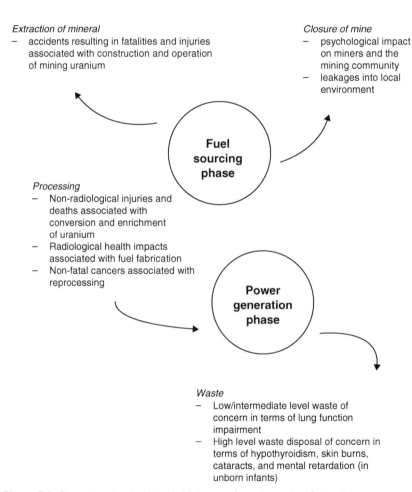

Figure 5.1 Occupational and public health impacts from the nuclear fuel cycle
Source: IIED (1999)

health at each stage. The nuclear fuel cycle has the potential for the greatest hazard due to the long half-life of the radionuclides and the dangers of an acute accident.

Figure 5.1 sums up the main occupational and public health effects at each stage of the cycle. The health effects are not only related to the radiation, but also to the hazards of general industrial work with accidents and stress-related illness. There may be psychological as well as physical effects on the population living in close proximity to any stage of the fuel cycle.

Energy use and the effect on the environment

The production and consumption of energy have the potential to cause pollution. Table 5.5 is a summary of environmental degradation associated with the main sources of energy that are used today. Every type of fuel used for energy production carries its own risks and benefits as well as direct and indirect environmental impacts. It is important to be aware of these when setting standards, and to allow discussion of alternatives.

Table 5.5 Summary table of energy-related environmental degradation

	Accession and processing	Transportation	Utilization
non-renewable			
petroleum products	seepage, burning of gas in oil fields	pipe leaks, oil slicks in oceans	air pollution leading to global climate change
solid fuels	mining overburden, quarries	coal dust	air pollution leading to global climate change; CO_2, particulates
nuclear power	uranium tailings		release of radioactive matter and heat; disposal of spent fuel rods
renewable			
hydroelectricity	dam and reservoir related problems		
biomass fuels	deforestation; soil erosion; flooding		air pollution; release of particulates and CO_2, leading to global climate change

Source: Adapted from Gupta and Asher (1998)

Energy and sustainable development

Fuel used for energy in houses, vehicles and factories often comes from great distances and is likely to have undergone several processing and transport stages. When communities are considering the use of new fuel sources, it is not just the economic cost that must be taken into account, but also any environmental impact and sustainability of sources.

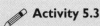

Activity 5.3

In order to reduce the impact of indoor air pollution in an area of India, it is proposed to encourage the use of kerosene for heating and cooking rather than the traditional wood fuel. What are the advantages and disadvantages to the environment and to health of using kerosene as opposed to wood? Consider not only the fuel itself, but also the method of harvesting or extraction and transport – in other words, the whole fuel cycle.

Feedback

According to the WHO (1997), wood burning for cooking and heating causes direct health effects from accidents and indoor air pollution, leading to respiratory problems; it mainly affects women and children. Kerosene burns more cleanly and the health impact seems clear when compared to wood, however, the fuel cycle is long:

- starting with an oil well in the Persian Gulf
- shipment across the Arabic Sea
- processing in a refinery in Bombay
- transport by train to the nearest state capital
- transport by truck to the village

There are environmental health impacts at each stage of the fuel cycle and there are costs from transport-related pollution and the risk of accidental spillage. In terms of air pollution, burning kerosene is cleaner than wood. However, when rest of the fuel cycle is included, this advantage is not as great as it first appears. Kerosene still carries a risk of fire and of poisoning. Another important consideration which is more difficult to quantify, is that of the security risk arising from dependence on petroleum imports; these are subject to political will and global events. On the other hand, the use of wood for fuel can lead to ecosystem disruption from over-harvesting and other risks. It is important to balance the different direct and indirect health effects of different fuel types as an essential part of long-term planning of energy use for sustainable development.

In order to be sustainable, energy consumption and production must balance environmental impact, social factors and economics. As discussed, issues surrounding energy production and consumption need to be addressed in high income as well as low and middle income countries, supplying enough energy for all at an affordable cost, both in economic and environmental terms. There are various ways in which a sufficient supply of energy for development can be met, first, by increasing energy production, and second, by using energy more efficiently. Examples of these include insulating homes to keep heat in and cold out and using energy-efficient lighting or burning biomass more efficiently in modified stoves. Changing fuels may also lead to energy efficiencies, for example, switching to electric rather than gasoline-driven modes of transport reduces pollution and the reliance on fossil fuel. Many countries rely heavily on imported fuels; fluctuations in oil prices can make the provision of affordable energy for all more difficult and can lead to the use of 'dirty' fuels such as biomass as an alternative; it can also lead to a decision to reduce energy use for heating. Both of these scenarios are detrimental to health.

Renewable energy and sustainable development

This chapter has mostly focused on non-renewable sources of energy, with the exception of hydroelectricity. Sustainable development and compliance with the Kyoto Protocol to reduce greenhouse gas emissions mean that there must be a greater reliance on the use of renewable sources in the future. Currently renewable sources account for only a fraction of world energy supply. New technology has allowed greater energy efficiency from renewable sources and is reducing the costs. Ethanol derived from the fermentation of biomass crops such as corn may eventually replace gasoline, a needed solution, as fossil fuels will eventually run out. Wind generation both on shore and offshore is the fastest-growing source of renewable energy. Denmark generates 20 per cent of its electricity from wind and in Europe overall 40 million people receive wind-generated electricity (Brown 2003). The production of cheap electricity from wind or hydroelectric plants may make it economical to produce hydrogen by the electrolysis of water. If hydrogen is utilized as an energy source in fuel cells, it is possible that in the future we may be able to power motor vehicles and supply electricity for heating, and cooling for buildings. Converting wind and hydroelectric energy into hydrogen is an easier method of storing and transporting fuel; it can be transported by pipeline or in liquefied form by ship for use in other locations. Many technical problems still need to be overcome in order to transport hydrogen safely. One way might be to transport 'interstitial' hydrogen stored within metals via roads.

In order to meet the Millennium Development Goals discussed at the beginning of the chapter, and to consider health effects when implementing a sustainable energy policy, it makes sense to increase the use of renewable energy sources, and to decrease the reliance upon those sources that need combustion to release their stored energy.

Summary

In this chapter, you will have seen some examples of how energy use and production impact significantly on the quality of the environment. The world's energy needs are growing; continuing economic development will inevitably lead to increased energy consumption and production. Environmental and health impacts from this vary, depending on the source of the energy and on the fuel cycle. All of these effects must be taken into account, along with local or global considerations, when any increase in energy production is contemplated, from any source. There are alternative ways of reducing these impacts such as by using renewable sources of energy; these may be essential to reduce the damage to the environment and achieve sustainable development.

References

Ahern M, Hunt A, Wilkinson P and Ebi KL (2004) Exposure and health impacts of electric power generation, transmission and distribution, in Menne B and Markandya A (eds) *Energy, Sustainable Development and Health*. Geneva: WHO.

Brown L (2003) Wind power set to become world's leading energy source: Earth Policy Institute. http://www.earth-policy.org/Updates/Update24.htm. Accessed 15 February 2005.

Chinese Embassy (2005) http://www.china-embassy.org/eng/zt/sxgc/t36512.htm. Accessed 15 February 2005.

Gupta A and Asher M (1998) *Environment and the Developing World.* Chichester: John Wiley and Sons.

IIED (1999) Final report – Mining, minerals and sustainable development. The results of a project for the World Business Council for Sustainable Development. London: International Institute for Environment and Development.

International Energy Agency (2004) *Energy Balances of Non-OECD Countries, 2001–2002.* Paris: IEA Publications.

IRN (2005) International Rivers Network: http://www.irn.org/. Accessed 15 February 2005.

Moeller DW (1997) *Environmental Health.* Cambridge, MA: Harvard University Press.

Pittman, AC (1998) Power generation and distribution, in Stellman JM (ed) *Environmental and Public Health Issues: Encyclopaedia of Occupational Health and Safety.* Geneva: International Labour Office, 3: 76.16–76.17.

UN (2004) Millennium Goals: http://www.un.org/millenniumgoals/. Accessed 10 May 2004.

WHO (1997) *Environment, Health and Sustainable Development.* Geneva: WHO.

Further reading

Chernobyl disaster: http://www.chernobyl.co.uk/

Energy sources: http://www.energy.gov/engine/content.do?BT_CODE=ENERGYSOURCES

Home energy audit: http://www.eere.energy.gov/consumerinfo/energy_savers/energyuse.html

Ministry of Non-conventional Energy Sources, Government of India: http://mnes.nic.in/

6 | **Waste**

Overview

The production of waste is a consequence of human activity. Waste is produced as a result of mining, energy production, or manufacturing and domestic activities. This waste is produced in a number of forms: air, liquid or solid, any of which may be hazardous. Each type of waste needs to be dealt with in the best practicable way in order to minimize its effects on the environment and on health. This chapter deals with a number of ways of defining and dealing with waste and considers in more detail how solid waste disposal can best be achieved in developing countries.

Learning objectives

By the end of this chapter, you will be better able to:

- **distinguish between the main types of waste and waste disposal strategies**
- **describe the main possible methods of human exposure to hazardous waste**
- **explain the potential health impacts of different waste disposal strategies**
- **understand global issues of waste management**

Key terms

Best Practical Environmental Option (BPEO) Identifies the preferred waste route in order to minimize harm and ensure the protection of the environment.

Bias Any error that results in a systematic deviation from the estimation of the allocation between exposure and outcome.

Confounding Situation in which an estimate of the association between a risk factor (exposure) and outcome is disturbed because of the association of the exposure with another risk factor (a confounding variable) for the outcome under study.

Landfill Method of solid waste disposal in which refuse is buried between layers of soil, or the site used for such disposal.

Waste hierarchy Methods of waste disposal from re-use (best environmental option) to disposal (worst).

Introduction to waste

Waste production is one of the major human activities affecting environmental quality. The exploitation of natural resources is driven by a society's need for socioeconomic development within the global market, and basic individual-level requirements to maintain a standard of living. These driving forces have increased the tendency of humans to exploit natural resources, with little or no regard to the quantity or quality of waste produced, or to the effects of this waste on local or global ecosystems. Socioeconomic development, driven by the exploitation of resources, has enabled a part of the global population to benefit from a higher quality of life. However, the remaining proportion of the global population, larger and more rapidly growing, must often over-exploit what are frequently already impoverished resources in order to satisfy their minimum needs. Therefore, actions that contribute to waste production are attributable to both poor and rich alike, and are a threat to the quality of life for future generations.

What is waste?

Waste is a material, substance or product that the owner no longer wants at a given place and time. There are a number of sources of waste: domestic, municipal, clinical, industrial, commercial and agricultural. Waste can also be defined according to the types of controls necessary to deal with it; these are known as controlled wastes, difficult wastes or hazardous wastes. These three categories of waste are disposed of in different ways, which attempt to minimize their impact on people and the environment.

When waste is defined according to its source, there are a number of different classifications of wastes which must be considered. For example, household wastes include all gases, liquids and solids generated by domestic activity which are discarded or emitted, of no immediate use to others. These wastes place great pressure on the environment and are closely linked to patterns of unsustainable consumption and production.

Waste can be broken down into sub-categories based on physical state: gaseous, liquid and solid. Table 6.1 gives some examples of solid wastes from different sources. You should note the variety of wastes from paper to construction debris and the presence of hazardous wastes.

As you can see in Table 6.1, all human activities generate waste, some contributing more than others. Figure 6.1 describes the waste generated by different sectors in European countries. Most of the waste is generated by mining and quarrying (29 per cent) and construction and demolition (22 per cent). Different strategies are appropriate for dealing with waste in each sector. For example, most of the waste from mining and quarrying remains at or near the site, whereas municipal waste is removed and dealt with in a number of ways, including recycling and disposal.

Table 6.1 Solid waste sources in Asia

Source	Typical waste generators	Types of solid wastes
Residential	Single and multifamily dwellings	Food wastes, paper, cardboard, plastics, textiles, leather, yard wastes, wood, glass, metals, ashes, special wastes (e.g., bulky items, consumer electronics, white goods, batteries, oil, tires), and household hazardous wastes
Industrial	Light and heavy manufacturing, fabrication, construction sites, power and chemical plants	Housekeeping wastes, packaging food wastes, construction and demolition materials, hazardous wastes, ashes, special wastes
Commercial	Stores, hotels, restaurants, markets, office buildings, etc.	Paper, cardboard, plastics, wood, food wastes, glass, metals, special wastes, hazardous wastes
Institutional	Schools, hospitals, prisons, government centers	Same as commercial
Construction and demolition	New construction sites, road repair, renovation sites, demolition of buildings	Wood, steel, concrete, dirt, etc.
Municipal services	Street cleaning, landscaping, parks, beaches, other recreational areas, water and wastewater treatment plants	Street sweepings; landscape and tree trimmings; general wastes from parks, beaches, and other recreational areas; sludge
Process	Heavy and light manufacturing, refineries, chemical plants, power plants, mineral extraction and processing	Industrial process wastes, scrap materials, off-specification products, slag, tailings
All of the above should be included as 'municipal solid waste'.		
Agriculture	Crops, orchards, vineyards, dairies, feedlots, farms	Spoiled food wastes, agricultural wastes, hazardous wastes (e.g., pesticides)

Source: World Bank Report (1999)

Public concern about environmental problems

The public are concerned about environmental issues, and in particular the fate of waste. Figure 6.2 describes public concern in the UK on environmental issues. Note that 95 per cent of respondents were concerned about chemicals entering water supplies. Until the 1970s there was very little concern over the selection of waste sites, and there was very little legislation in the UK or elsewhere to control and monitor the disposal of waste materials which might present a hazard to human health. Waste was dumped in the nearest convenient place, such as a disused mineshaft, quarry or local stream. This practice still occurs in regions or countries without controls or a waste management strategy that is not enforced.

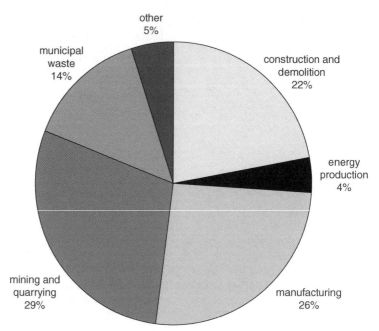

Figure 6.1 Total waste generation by sector: EEA Countries 1992–97
Source: Eurostat

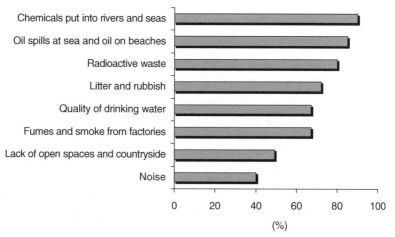

Figure 6.2 Public concern over environmental issues
Source: Office for National Statistics (1999)

There were some high profile cases concerning hazardous waste dumps in the 1970s which focused public attention on the possible health implications, for example, the Love Canal waste dump. Love Canal is situated in New York State, USA. From the 1930s to the 1950s, 20,000 tonnes of hazardous materials were dumped here and buried in landfill. The land was then sold on for development, and houses were built on the site in the 1950s and the 1960s. By the 1970s complaints of ill health were being reported. The site was found to be causing contamination of air, soil and water by leaking waste. The residents had to be evacuated and the leaks contained. Some of the health effects reported included low birth weight, a high incidence of birth defects, seizures and learning problems (Brown and Clapp 2002). There is a follow-up study currently underway to examine the longer-term health effects.

Health risks from waste sites, even those containing hazardous materials, are difficult to study and to quantify. This chapter will offer an introduction to some of the issues surrounding waste and the varied pathways to environmental and health problems.

How much waste?

The USA is the biggest producer of waste world-wide with over six billion tonnes per year. Although it makes up only 4.6 per cent of the world's population, the USA produces 33 per cent of the world's solid waste.

Comparing wastes between countries can be difficult as different definitions of waste might be used. For instance, municipal solid waste may or may not include demolition and construction waste. In the USA, much of the solid waste generated is from mining activities and is largely unregulated. In Asia, urban waste is two to three times that of rural areas, although it is difficult to measure the volume of rural waste as it may be dumped in isolated areas or incinerated domestically. Figure 6.3 summarizes the types of solid waste from high, middle and low income countries. The types of waste differ, with organic waste dominating in middle and low income countries and large volumes of paper waste in high income countries.

Waste management

Sustainable development is based on meeting the goals and needs of the present generation without compromising the needs of future generations. Therefore, it is not appropriate simply to keep disposing of waste in various, unmanaged ways. Clear methods for waste management need to be in place, determining how to reduce it or process it in the best practicable way. The treatment of waste is defined as any method, technique, or process that is designed to change the physical, chemical, or biological character or composition of a (hazardous) waste. Ideally this will act to neutralize it, recover unexploited energy, render it less hazardous or make it safer to transport, store or dispose of.

The waste hierarchy

The concept of waste management for sustainable development is based on the waste hierarchy. Priority is placed on the re-use and recycling of waste rather than its disposal. The waste hierarchy (Figure 6.4) can be used as a guide to help ensure an integrated approach to waste management policy or decision making. Each decision is based on the most environmentally sound way to deal with waste.

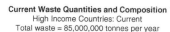

Current Waste Quantities and Composition
High Income Countries: Current
Total waste = 85,000,000 tonnes per year

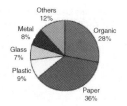

2025 Waste Quantities and Composition
High Income Countries: Year 2025
Total waste = 86,000,000 tonnes per year

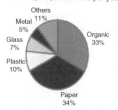

Middle Income Countries: Current
Total waste = 34,000,000 tonnes per year

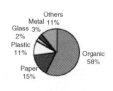

Middle Income Countries: Year 2025
Total waste = 111,000,000 tonnes per year

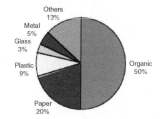

Low Income Countries: Current
Total waste = 158,000,000 tonnes per year

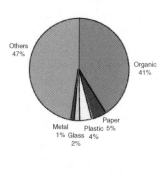

Low Income Countries: Year 2025
Total waste = 480,000,000 tonnes per year

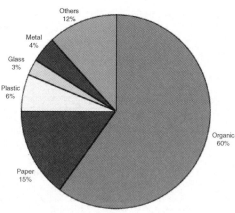

Note: Approximate scale only

Figure 6.3 Waste types in high income and low income countries
Source: World Bank (1999)

This requires information on: the nature of the waste; legislative issues; environmental impacts and the technical feasibility of the options. The costs and benefits of each option can also be calculated. The aim should be to focus on the best environmental option. For example, a product can be designed in such a way that when it is dismantled it optimizes the potential of the material primarily through re-use or recycling. Many countries are now using financial and legislative measures, such as Landfill Taxes and the Packaging Regulations to target local

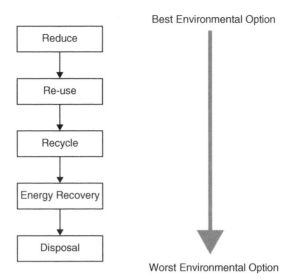

Figure 6.4 Waste hierarchy

authorities and those responsible for municipal and industrial waste. The aim is to reduce the amount of rubbish and encourage recycling and waste minimization. The same incentive works for consumers. Where consumers have to pay for each bag of rubbish produced, they reduce the amount they dispose of and recycle or compost materials that would otherwise be thrown away.

Future strategies for waste disposal encourage the disposal of waste as near to its place of production as possible (proximity principle). Another concept is the 'Best Practical Environmental Option (BPEO)'. This may be described as a systematic and consultative decision-making procedure which emphasizes the protection and conservation of the environment across land, air and water. The United Kingdom has a waste management strategy that is based on these three principles: waste hierarchy, BPEO and the proximity principle (DEFRA 2004).

Waste prevention/minimization

This is a key factor in any waste management strategy. Waste prevention aims to reduce the amount of waste generated in the first place. By reducing or removing altogether the presence of hazardous substances in waste materials, it also leads to a simplification of disposal practices. Waste prevention is closely linked with improvements in the manufacturing process and is influenced by public opinion, for example, by consumer demand for 'greener' products which might use less packaging. Adapting industrial processes can eliminate or reduce emissions, for example, by removing lead solders from electronic products, the pollution associated with manufacture as well as disposal at the end of the product's useful life will be reduced. Waste can also be decreased by using products that are designed to last longer and be easier to repair or recycle.

Industries in many high income countries are realizing that waste minimization can improve efficiency and reduce costs, helping in turn to reduce waste produced at the household level. In these countries, the promotion of waste minimization as a target has been hampered due to a lack of data on waste production at source, and on facilities for waste collection and disposal.

Methods of recycling and re-use

At the end of a product's life, as many of the component materials as possible should be recovered for re-use or recycling. Several 'waste streams' have been ear-marked for special concern. These include: packaging waste; end-of-life vehicles; batteries; electrical and electronic waste. Several European Union countries are already managing to recycle over 50 per cent of packaging.

Recycling and re-use appear to be practical solutions for waste management. There are three main factors that hinder recycling. The first is that the cost to the consumer at market price does not include the costs to the environment or health, nor the costs of the raw materials. The second factor is that there are more tax/other financial incentives for the extraction of raw materials than for recycling industries; the last factor is the lack of markets for recycled materials. There are moves to encourage recycling and re-use in different countries, particularly in relation to plastic packaging wastes.

Recycling

There are two types of recycling: the first is primary or closed-loop recycling, where post-consumer materials such as glass, paper, metals and plastics are collected and recycled to create new products of the same type; for instance, newspapers into newspapers, aluminium soft drink cans into aluminium soft drink cans. This method can reduce the use of virgin materials in a product by 20–90 per cent. The other type of recycling is secondary or open-loop recycling and reduces the use of virgin material by 25 per cent; in this system the waste material is converted into different products, for example, polypropylene ice-cream containers or straws are re-manufactured as clothes pegs or rubbish bins. Recycling often uses less energy than waste disposal and conserves resources as well as preventing waste from ending up in landfill or incinerators. Recycling does still produce pollution, but the emissions are generally lower than those produced by using virgin sources in manufacturing. For recycling to work effectively, there has to be an incentive for the consumer, such as ease of recycling, or payment for collection of other rubbish that is not recyclable.

Re-use

Products can be designed to be used a number of times before becoming obsolete. For example, food and drink containers or car tyres can be designed to be re-usable. Products can be re-used (or repaired) by another consumer and they can also be specifically designed to make re-use or recycling simpler by changing the components or method of construction or manufacture. Goods can be re-used at a consumer level by finding new uses for them, such as using plastic shopping bags as rubbish bin liners.

The advantages of re-use are savings in energy and raw materials, reduced disposal needs and costs and cost savings for businesses and consumers. There are also new market opportunities available, for example, refillable products. For re-use to work, there needs to be interaction and communication between producers and consumers and communication of consumer needs.

Composting

A large percentage of municipal waste (92 per cent in Karachi and 26 per cent in New York City) is biodegradable and suitable for composting. Composting can be achieved by individuals at home or by 'community composting' schemes. Composting removes waste from landfill or incineration and creates a product that can then be used again as a soil nutrient, mulch or cover for completed landfill sites. It is also useful for restoring eroded land and improving agricultural soil. Community composting plants are not without concerns; they may leach into water sources or produce gaseous emissions (mainly carbon dioxide and methane). Workers may be exposed to pathogenic fungi and bacteria and organic waste may contain toxic substances.

Waste water

Waste water can also be recycled. For example, the development of facilities to re-use grey water (waste water from washing and domestic appliances) would significantly cut the amounts of fresh water used for such activities as toilet flushing or car washing.

Improving final disposal and monitoring

The way in which waste is finally disposed of is of major concern to society and to the practice of sustainability. In many countries, wastes of all types are all buried together in a landfill. This practice may have a number of deleterious effects on the environment, on human health and on the quality of life. Waste that cannot be recycled or re-used should be safely incinerated and landfill should only be used as a last resort. Both methods of disposal have the potential to cause harm to people and the environment, particularly if the landfill sites or incinerators are poorly regulated. In many high income countries, there are strict guidelines in place for landfill and incineration. The use of recycling, landfill, and incineration as disposal options varies greatly by country, even within the high income countries of Europe.

Hazardous waste

Some waste falls into a special category known as hazardous waste. There are different regulations in place relating to this type of waste and the means of its disposal. A large variety of waste has the potential to be hazardous if not handled in a satisfactory manner. There is no unified agreement on what can be specifically called 'hazardous wastes', but a useful definition given by the British Medical Association (BMA 1991) is that hazardous wastes 'have the potential to cause harm to human health and the environment if they are improperly treated, stored, transported, or inadequately disposed of'.

The waste can be described by its properties by the industry or technology of origin, by specific constituents, or a combination of these. There are some other definitions that are used to describe hazardous wastes, for instance, in the UK they are sometimes referred to as 'special wastes' or 'difficult wastes'.

Solid waste management in different countries

The practice of solid waste management varies from country to country, depending on many factors, including the resources available. Waste management varies between high and low income countries. The main difference is in organization, for instance, there is a formalized process of collection of waste in high income countries, contrasting with informal or erratic collections in low and middle income countries. Another difference is in the use of resources and technology (Table 6.2).

 Activity 6.1

 1 What do you think are the barriers for low income countries managing solid waste?
 2 What are the opportunities for low income countries to reduce waste using the experiences of middle and high income countries as an example?

 Feedback

 1 The main barriers for the management of solid waste in low income countries are cost, the availability of technology, space for landfill, and dealing with the increasing and changing volumes of waste that appear as countries develop, for example, growing amounts of paper waste and disposable items such as food containers.

 2 Low income countries have the opportunity to learn from the mistakes and successes of other countries in dealing with solid municipal waste, for instance, encouraging community participation and composting at local level. Low income countries typically have a high volume of organic waste without the capacity for households to be able to deal with this waste themselves. Better technologies are now available to enable small-scale efficient incineration projects. Low income countries can formalize the practice of re-use and recycling that already works well informally. To achieve economic sustainability of waste disposal, an improved fee collection system could be put into place – following middle income country examples of best practice.

Health effects of waste disposal

There are a number of methods of waste disposal available, each with its advantages and disadvantages and differing impacts on health and the environment. If waste substances are volatile, it is likely that vapours will be released from a landfill into

Table 6.2 Comparison of typical solid waste management practices in low, middle and high income countries

Activity	Low income	Middle income	High income
Source reduction	No organized programmes, but re-use and low per capita waste generation are common	Discussion of source reduction is rarely incorporated in organized programmes	Organized programmes beginning to emphasize source reduction and re-use of materials
Collection	Sporadic and inefficient; service limited to high visibility area and wealthy businesses willing to pay	Improved service and increased collection from residential areas. Larger vehicle fleet and some mechanization	Collection rate greater than 90 per cent. Compactor trucks and mechanized vehicles are common
Landfill	Low technology sites; usually open dumping	Some controlled and sanitary landfills with environmental controls. Still some open dumping	Sanitary landfills with a combination of liners, leak detection, leachate and gas detection and treatment systems
Incineration	Not common or successful as there are high capital and operating costs. Problems are caused by high moisture content in the waste and high percentage of inert material	Some incinerators used, but with financial and operating difficulties	Prevalent in areas with high land costs. Most have some form of environmental controls and energy recovery system
Recycling	Mostly through informal sector and waste picking. Mainly localized markets and imports of materials for recycling	Informal sector still involved. Some high technology sorting and processing facilities. Materials may be imported for recycling	Recyclable material collection services and high technology sorting and processing facilities. Increasing attention to long-term markets
Composting	Rarely undertaken, even though waste stream has a high organic component	Large composting units are generally unsuccessful; some smaller projects are sustainable	Increasing in popularity for backyard and large-scale facilities. Waste stream has a smaller proportion of biodegradable content
Costs	Collection costs represent 90 per cent of the municipal solid waste budget; waste fees regulated by some local governments but fee collection system is inefficient	Collection costs are 50–80 per cent of the budget. Waste fees are regulated by some local and national governments, more innovation for fee collection	Collection costs are less than 10 per cent of the budget. Large budget allocations to intermediate waste treatment facilities. Upfront community participation reduces costs and increases options available to waste planners (e.g. recycling and composting)

Source: Adapted from World Bank (1999)

the air. Incineration may destroy such substances but combustion is well known to create toxic substances such as sulphur dioxide (SO_2), oxides of nitrogen (NO_x), polychlorinated biphenyls (PCBs) and dioxins. Composting can also generate hazardous substances, for example, some of the micro-organisms which flourish in the composting process are able to release spores with allergenic properties which can stimulate or exacerbate respiratory diseases. Even recycling processes are not without their risks. These may well involve the expenditure of energy and the consequent release of combustion gases or contaminated wash waters.

Studies on the health effects of waste disposal are specific to each disposal or management method used, as each method of waste management is likely to give rise to different pollutants and different exposure routes (Figure 6.5). The difficulties in assessing the health effects of waste disposal not only arise from methodological issues (such as measuring exposure and health outcomes; study design; control of confounding factors, and statistical power) but also in many cases from the sheer paucity of available human epidemiological studies. Toxicological data may be available for specific contaminants but provide limited information on the likely human health impact of a complex environmental pollution source such as a waste site.

Landfill

To create a site that is suitable for landfill, a number of factors have to be taken into consideration such as the location of the site and its geology and hydro-geology. For example, are there drinking water boreholes nearby? Is it situated on a flood-plain or in wetlands, and so on? Landfill sites can also act as breeding grounds for pests like rats which may in turn be vectors for human diseases. The next factor is the design and engineering of the site. The site may aim to use dilution (mixing waste from different sources) and dispersal, or rely on containment (keeping the waste from air, soil or water outside the site). Will there be co-disposal – dealing with hazardous waste at the same time as domestic or other waste? It is crucial to keep these forms of waste from re-entering the environment and so disposal methods need to consider how reducing leachate and gas formation can be achieved, and to ensure protection against flooding. The operation of the site needs to be taken into account; how will the waste be covered or capped; what is the access to the site; who will have access and how will it be monitored? Such considerations may lead to extra road construction. The site has to be monitored to ensure its safe operation and this also applies when it has been decommissioned. The key factor for human health when related to landfill is not what goes *into* the site, but what comes *out*.

Used tyres are a huge waste problem. They have been dumped in landfill and in illegal sites and may be breeding grounds for mosquitoes and a fire risk. Once a fire has started in a tyre dump, it is extremely difficult to extinguish and is a source of toxic air pollution and water run-off.

There are a number of ways to prevent tyres from entering landfill. Some tyres are suitable for re-treading and using again. They can be filled with soil and used as foundations and walls in low-cost solar homes (although they should be sealed to prevent air pollutants). Some have been used to form artificial reefs to attract fish.

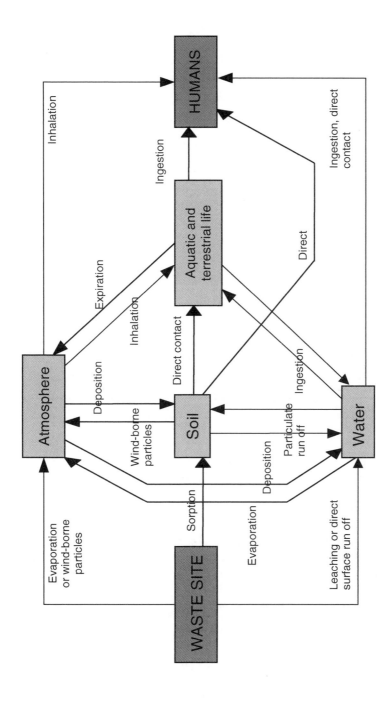

Figure 6.5 Exposure routes from waste to humans

They have been used to build walls to reduce noise along highways. They can be recycled and used to make resins for car bumpers, doormats, and road building materials.

Tyres have a higher heating value per unit of weight than coal and can be less polluting; they can be used to generate electrics or to fuel cement kilns.

Landfill – assessing health effects

The main problem with assessing health effects from landfill is determining the exposure to human health. There are three main problems with this:

- unknown mixture of chemicals (what is in the landfill? There may be some information available if it is an official hazardous waste site.)
- unknown exposure route (air, water, soil, agricultural products)
- unknown dose (how much of each chemical).

There have been single and multi-site studies that have a found a number of different health outcomes that are weakly or strongly associated with living near to landfill sites. Table 6.3 gives some examples and an estimation of the strength of the association. The problem with all of the studies is the lack of exposure data and the small numbers involved. A study looking at over 9,000 landfill sites in the UK gives some more detailed evidence, although it is still an ecological study. There was no increase in cancer; a 1 per cent increase in congenital anomalies, rising to 7 per cent when near to hazardous sites and a 5 per cent increase in low birth weight (Elliott et al. 2001).

Table 6.3 Strength of health effects found around landfill studies

Health effect	Strength
Self-reported health symptoms: headaches, fatigue, sleepiness[1]	++
Low birth weight	+++/–
Birth defects	++/–
Cancer	+/– –

Note: [1] due to toxic chemicals, stress and fears or a reporting bias?

There are biases and confounding factors in these studies which can explain some of the effects, but the evidence seems to suggest that they may indicate some real risks associated with residence near some types of landfill sites. Despite a substantial number of studies conducted, risks to health from landfill sites are still hard to quantify, as there is often insufficient exposure information and the effects of low-level exposure in the general population are difficult to establish.

Incineration

Waste disposal using incineration is the process of burning waste through the use of incinerators, industrial boilers, furnaces, kilns or other facilities. Incineration reduces the volume of waste by about 90 per cent, a significant reduction of waste that would otherwise go into a landfill. Of course the solid waste left after incineration must be disposed of in landfill facilities. Incineration at high temperatures also destroys many of the toxics and pathogens in medical and other hazardous wastes. Not only can it be used to get rid of waste, but also as a method of energy recovery and heat generation.

Incineration – the main concerns

Incineration produces pollutants which are derived from three sources; they are present in waste feed (or its precursor); they are formed in the combustion process (for instance, through incomplete oxidation) and they are created by reformation reactions in gas cooling or air pollution control devices. They are released as air pollution which may contain dioxins, heavy metals (cadmium, mercury and lead,) acid gases (NO_x, SO_x, HCl) and particulates, all of which are harmful to human and ecosystem health. The other source of pollution is the resultant ash. Bottom ash is left at the end of the process; this can contain toxic material and methods of disposal for this are of concern. In low-polluting incinerators, the solid ash can be used as a mix with cement for building blocks or paths. For incinerators dealing with hazardous substances, the solid ash has to be dumped in specially designated landfill sites. The type and concentration of contaminants will depend on the process type, the waste being burned and the combustion conditions.

Incineration – health effects

The health effects of incineration are found in two main populations: the local residents and workers at the incinerator plants. There is some evidence in the literature to suggest that workers are exposed to higher concentrations of dioxins and toxic metals than in other forms of employment and that this might lead to health consequences. There have been few studies of residents near incinerators and pollution-related ill health may be difficult to detect. Looking at small populations, low concentrations of those pollutants causing concern and long latency periods for effect from some pollutants compound these difficulties.

Based on the known individual pollutants from incineration, it is possible to estimate the likely health effects associated with the process. These include:

- dioxins: cancers, birth defects
- heavy metals: range of health effects (acute toxicity, cancer, reproductive effects)
- particulates: mortality, respiratory disease.

The Committee on Health Effects of Waste Incineration (2000) assessed the health effects from pollutants in incinerators using MACT (maximum achievable control technology). They concluded that workers have the greatest risk and those living near a single facility have a small risk. Table 6.4 provides further detail.

Table 6.4 Potential health effects from an efficient incinerator

Substance	Potential effects on workers at a facility	Potential effects from a single facility on a local population	Potential effects from multiple facilities on a broader population
Particulate matter	Substantial	minimal	minimal
Dioxins	Substantial	minimal	substantial
Lead	Substantial	minimal	moderate
Mercury	Substantial	minimal	moderate
Other metals	Substantial	minimal	moderate
Acidic gases	Moderate	negligible	negligible
Acidic aerosols	Moderate	minimal	minimal

Source: Committee on Health Effects of Waste Incineration (2000)

Global issues of waste management

Climate change

All waste management options have some impact on climate change. Landfill sites produce methane gas (CH_4) which contributes to global warming in the atmosphere. Incineration leads to the production of another greenhouse gas, carbon dioxide (CO_2), although waste-to-energy incineration reduces the need for more polluting fossil fuels. Recycling can also contribute to climate change as it uses energy (fossil fuels). The production process, however, is less energy-intensive than using primary sources. Composting also emits carbon dioxide and methane. Reduction and re-use have a generally positive impact although the issue of transport of goods for recycling, re-use and composting must be taken into account. It is here that the proximity principle (that waste should be dealt with close to its source) is important when reducing the contribution of waste disposal to climate change.

Sustainable waste management limits the increase of the greenhouse effect and the enlargement of the ozone hole; it reduces acidic precipitation, deforestation, desertification and the loss of biodiversity.

Transportation

A further issue of global waste management is the trans-boundary movement of wastes – either as air or water pollution, or as the physical transfer of wastes (often hazardous) for reprocessing or storage in another country.

Waste picking in low and middle income countries

There are special considerations surrounding waste management in low and middle income countries. The health impacts of waste that is not collected (including injury, intoxication, infection) can affect the vulnerable in a community. In some areas, micro-economies develop that are based on the picking over of waste (whether collected or not) and selling on any reusable or recyclable material. The health of these waste pickers – often children – is of concern and is the subject of a number of studies and initiatives to improve their circumstances.

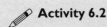 **Activity 6.2**

Read the extract by Selvam (1994) and then give a summary of how Panaji hopes to achieve an efficient and sustainable waste management system.

 An example of an integrated waste management system in a developing country

Panaji, the capital of Goa, is a small but well-developed town with a population of 42,915. Panaji Municipal Council (PMC) is responsible for the collection, transportation and disposal of solid wastes generated within the municipal limits. Households and establishments including hospitals, private nursing homes, restaurants, etc., deposit their wastes in communal waste storage bins, for subsequent collection (manual) and transportation to an undeveloped and unsanitary dumping site. A large number of waste pickers make their livelihood by collecting a variety of recyclable wastes from bins and the disposal site. Households (40 per cent) and restaurants (27 per cent) are the two major waste generators. About 1.8 tons, 8 per cent of total wastes, are collected daily by waste pickers for recycling.

The major issues raised by the community are: inadequate number and faulty design of bins, irregular clearing by PMC workers, and the wet and unhygienic conditions around the bins. Meetings with representatives of other major waste generators, restaurants, hospitals and nursing homes revealed their preference for a personalized 'door-to-door' system and their willingness to pay for the improved service level.

The social survey findings formed an important basis for the development of a sustainable solid waste management model. For example, the Panaji survey provided some unexpected results; people in Panaji are not interested in 'door-to-door' collection of wastes; people are willing to make a monthly payment of Rs.10/- (US$ 1 = INR 31.80 6/94 rate) per household for a communal primary waste collection system with an improved bin design and daily clearance through a mechanized system.

Various disposal options such as composting, pelletization, incineration, etc. were evaluated. The potential for resource recovery and revenue generation influenced the decision for composting organic wastes from vegetable markets and restaurants.

Recommendations to improve the existing solid waste management situation:

- Replace the existing bottomless cement concrete bins with suitable numbers of metallic bins, a minimum of one bin within 50 m of all households.
- Collect the restaurant wastes from 'door-to-door', twice a day, on a full cost recovery basis. The six existing closed body vehicles should be used for servicing 200 restaurants per day.
- Collect the infectious wastes separately from hospitals and nursing homes for incineration at the Goa Government Medical College Hospital, on a full cost recovery basis.
- Use the existing garbage compactor exclusively for collecting the organic wastes from the municipal market.

Waste disposal:

- Install a manual composting plant for processing eight tons of restaurant and market wastes everyday. With proper marketing, it is not only possible to fully recover the production cost of Rs. 325/- per ton, but also possible to make a modest profit.
- Develop the abandoned laterite stone quarry pit into a sanitary landfill site. Improve the existing dump site operation (until the new site is developed) by spreading the waste and covering it with construction wastes using a hired bulldozer on a regular basis.
- Sustain the waste pickers', contribution to resource recovery, by organizing them into a formal group with the help of a local NGO, providing them with tools to sort out wastes, raising their status to that of waste collectors, and providing either free or low-cost medical facilities through the state health department.

 Feedback

In order to be sustainable, the waste management scheme has to include all aspects of waste, from production to disposal. This strategy did not cover waste prevention, but did propose a cost-effective method of dealing with waste after consultation with businesses and communities. Consumers are prepared to pay to have a more efficient and hygienic service. Composting will make a profit and waste pickers will have improved livelihoods. The local authority was able to ensure that resources were used effectively and that the system maximized waste collection and its subsequent recycling or disposal.

Summary

Waste is produced as the result of domestic and industrial activity. There are a number of ways to deal with waste, including reduction, recycling, minimization and disposal. The waste hierarchy can help to establish the best and most environmentally efficient method for dealing with waste, leaving disposal as the least preferred option. Disposal methods have the potential to harm both the environment and human health if not properly designed or maintained. The study of waste on human health is complicated by the difficulties of establishing exposure routes and the often unknown nature of the contaminants.

References

BMA (1991) *Hazardous Waste and Human Health*. Oxford: Oxford University Press.

Brown P and Clapp R. (2002) Looking back on Love Canal. *Public Health Report* 117(2): 95–8.

Committee on Health Effects of Waste Incineration (2000) *Waste Incineration and Public Health*. Washington, DC: National Academy Press.

DEFRA (2004) *Waste Implementation Programme: One Year on*. London: DEFRA.

Elliott P, Briggs D, Morris S et al. (2001) Risk of adverse birth outcomes in populations living near landfill sites. *British Medical Journal* 323(7309): 363–8.

Eurostat, EEA on specific waste streams: http://dataservice.eea.eu.int/atlas/viewdata/ viewpub.asp?id=392. Accessed 20 June 2005.

Office for National Statistics (1999) www.statistics.gov.uk

Selvam P (1994) Community-based SWM project preparation, 20th WEDC Conference, Colombo, Sri Lanka.

World Bank (1999) What a waste: solid waste management in Asia: www.worldbank.org/html/ fpd/urban/publicat/whatawaste.pdf

Further reading

Gupta S (2004) Rethinking waste management: www.indiatogether.org/2004/apr/ env-rethink.htm

South West Public Health Observatory (Waste Management and Public Health): http://www.swpho.org.uk/waste/impact_health.htm

Vrijheid M (2000) Health effects of residence near hazardous waste landfill sites: a review of epidemiologic literature. *Environmental Health Perspective* 108 (Suppl 1): 101–12.

World Bank Urban Solid Waste Management Sourcebook: http://www.worldbank.org/urban/ usolid waste management/

7 | Water and sanitation

Overview

Water, sanitation, and their relationship to health are crucial environmental health issues, especially so in low and middle income countries. This chapter will concentrate on the situation in low and middle income countries, although comparisons will be made with industrialized nations. Improving the water supply and sanitation in low and middle income countries will have a greater impact than in high income countries, as the prevailing conditions there are worse.

Learning objectives

By the end of this chapter, you will be better able to:

- **describe the importance of availability of water of sufficient quantity and quality**
- **explain the nature and extent of water-borne diseases**
- **give examples of major sources of water contamination**
- **give examples of the health consequences of inappropriate excreta disposal**
- **evaluate different criteria associated with standard-setting in relation to water supply**

Key terms

Eutrophication The enrichment of an ecosystem by plant nutrients, leading to possible new species change, decreased biodiversity, and toxicity.

Peri-urban On the urban margins.

Water-based disease Caused by disease-causing agents that spend part of their life cycle inside an intermediate aquatic host.

Water-borne disease Caused by the transmission of disease in drinking water.

Water-related vector-borne diseases Diseases spread by insects that either breed in water, or are found nearby.

Water scarcity Not enough water to supply all users' needs.

Water-washed Diseases which could be prevented through provision of increased quantities of water.

Access to water

Access to water is a fundamental human need, but according to the UN a third of the world's population live in countries with moderate to high 'water stress'. An area is experiencing water stress when annual water supplies drop below 1,700 m^3 per person.

'Water scarcity' occurs when the annual water supplies drop below 1,000 m^3 per person. Then the amount of water withdrawn from lakes, rivers or groundwater is so great that supplies are no longer adequate to satisfy all human or ecosystem requirements, resulting in increased competition between water users.

Access to water is not equitable. Those with the poorest access to adequate supplies of safe water tend to be communities who are already disadvantaged by poverty, such as those in peri-urban and rural areas. However, living in urban areas with adequate supplies of water available does not guarantee access; easy access to water often only reaches certain segments of the community.

In high income countries, the primary concern is the quality of the water supply. This can only be a relevant concern for the population if there is a sufficient quantity of water to supply people's basic needs. It has been estimated that 50 litres a day are required to supply the basic requirements of an individual (Table 7.1).

Table 7.1 Basic water requirements for human needs

Purpose	Litres/person/day
Drinking water	5
Sanitation	20
Bathing	15
Food preparation	10
Total	50

Source: Adapted from Gleick (1996)

Quality as well as quantity of water can be of serious concern. Water pollution (impairing quality) adds to the problem of supplying sufficient quantities because this effectively removes some of the viable water supply. An adequate water supply is essential not just for drinking and bathing, but for irrigation of crops, industry, generation of electricity, provision of sanitation and the supply of fish for food.

Table 7.2 shows the wide variety of demands on the water supply, and the quality of water required for each. High water quality is only needed for drinking and cooking (potable water). The other uses for water rely on having a sufficient quantity of water; quality is less important.

Table 7.2 The uses for water and the quality of water required for each

Use	Desirable quality for use	Quality after use
Water for consumption (potable water)	high quality; must meet predetermined standards	needs treatment
Water for hygiene and sanitation	high quality not required	needs treatment
General municipal use, fire fighting, street-cleaning, etc.	high quality not required; many cities use the potable water supply to avoid complication	needs treatment

Continued

Table 7.2 *Continued*

Use	Desirable quality for use	Quality after use
Generation of electricity	low sediment; usually uses dammed water	reusable; there is no change to the water
Industrial	low in sediment, mineral and biological contaminants	mostly reusable after treatment; could be very polluted, or of high temperature if not treated
Agriculture	not too saline or too alkaline	polluted by pesticides, herbicides, fertilizers and salts, needs treatment for immediate re-use

Source: Adapted from Gupta and Asher (1998)

 Activity 7.1

You have read about the importance of having access to a suitable quantity of water for drinking, sanitation and hygiene. Many people take access to water for granted. Consider the implications of having restricted access to water, describing the potential situation at your home if you have a household supply of water:

- How many taps do you have per person?
- How many flushable lavatories are there per person?

Monitor your household's use of water for a day; note how many times you turn on a tap or use appliances that consume water, such as flushing the lavatory. What is the water being used for? Try to restrict yourself to one tap – preferably the one furthest away from your kitchen, outside the house if possible. Try to restrict your use of water. Consider having to do this every day and supply enough for your family and possibly to irrigate crops.

If you don't have a household supply of water, consider how you get your water, who carries it and how the water is used.

 Feedback

This simple activity shows how access to water can be taken for granted by those for whom it is readily available. Each household will use water in different ways and so the answers you supply will vary considerably.

Time taken to access sufficient water

It is important to have a clear definition of what constitutes 'access to water'. Many statistics use the baseline for access as having a standpipe within 100 metres of a dwelling. If all of the water for a family of six people, i.e. 300 litres, has to be carried, this will require many trips to ensure adequate supply, which is both time-consuming and tiring.

The journey time to collect the water, both in distance and time spent in queues has a significant effect on water consumption (see Figure 7.1). It is mostly women and children who are involved in water collection; freeing women from this task allows them to spend more time in other essential tasks such as improving the family income, caring for children and preparing food. There is also a reduction in ill health and injury caused by transporting the water.

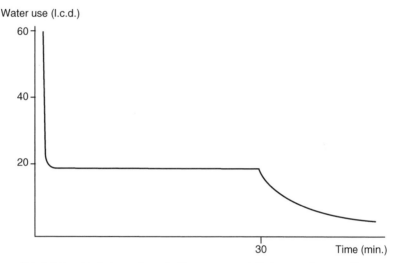

Figure 7.1 Relationship between household water use and the journey time to collect water
Source: Cairncross and Feachem (1993)

Water, health and disease

Faecal contamination is the world's leading environmental health problem. Over three million deaths a year are attributable to diarrhoea that could be avoided through adequate water supplies, sanitation and domestic hygiene. Chemical contamination of water, despite its dramatic media coverage, does not have the same health impact. The main diseases associated with water and sanitation are summarized in Table 7.3; they are responsible for millions of deaths and DALYs (disability adjusted life years) every year.

Water affects transmission of disease in four main ways, described as:

• water-borne
• water-washed
• water-based
• water-related.

Water-borne disease; faecal-oral

There are a number of different transmission routes that allow faecal contamination to spread. This has theoretical and practical implications for both

Table 7.3 Global burden of water and sanitation-related disease

	Mortality estimates for 2002	DALYs 2002
Water-borne (Faecal-oral)		
Diarrhoeal disease	1 798 000	61 966 000
Poliomyelitis	1 000	151 000
Water-washed		
Trachoma	<1000	2 329 000
Water-based		
Schistosomiasis	15 000	1 702 000
Water-related vector		
Malaria	1 272 000	46 496 000
Lymphatic filariasis	<1000	5 777 000
Dengue	19 000	616 000
Intestinal nematode infections (Helminths)	12 000	2 951 000

Source: WHO World Health Report (2002)

epidemiological understanding and disease control. It is difficult to identify the significance of a single transmission route, for example, drinking water, without understanding the role of the other routes such as food, flies, and unwashed fingers and so on, as shown in Figure 7.2.

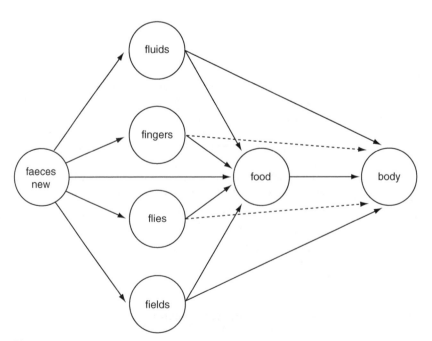

Figure 7.2 Transmission of disease from faeces

Source: Wagner and Lanoix (1958)

Preventative strategies include hygiene education to attempt to break cycles of transmission. It is also important to separate the public and private domains of water transmission. If the water supply in the public domain is contaminated with cholera, there is likely to be an epidemic. However, if the water supply is improved, it will not mean that disease is eradicated if transmission continues in the domestic situation, through open defecation, for instance.

Intestinal helminthic infections (worms)

Helminthic infections are related to sanitation rather than water supply, however, the transmission of the infection can be reduced by promotion of good hygiene when there is a sufficient water supply. The three most common infections are *Ascaris* (roundworm), *Trichuris* (whipworm) and *Necator* (hookworm). The first two are spread via the faecal to oral route and hookworms penetrate through the feet after the eggs have developed in moist soil. The biggest health burden from helminths is secondary to their contribution to malnutrition, growth retardation and lethargy. While there are many cases, few people die directly from these diseases.

Water-washed disease

These are diseases (such as skin and eye infections) which could be prevented through providing increased quantities of water. The leading example of this kind of disease is trachoma, which is the consequence of eye infection with *Chlamydia trachomatis*.

Trachoma is endemic in 49 countries, mostly in Africa, but also in the Eastern Mediterranean, South-East Asia and the Western Pacific. It remains the most common preventable cause of blindness in the world. There are an estimated 5.6 million people globally who are blind, visually impaired or at immediate risk of blindness from the disease and a further 146 million cases of active trachoma in need of treatment. Trachoma is common in areas of the world that are socio-economically deprived of basic needs in housing, health, water and sanitation. Having adequate quantities of water for washing can decrease numbers of infections by a median reduction of 25 per cent (Esrey et al. 1991).

Water-based disease

Infections are spread either through skin penetration (schistosomiasis), or through ingestion (guinea worm). The disease-causing agents of both spend part of their life cycle inside an intermediate aquatic host; the parasites spend some of their life cycle in humans, and some inside another water-based animal.

Schistosomiasis

The schistosomiasis parasite spends part of its life cycle inside snails; it then emerges into water and is able to penetrate the skin of people who are bathing or in contact with the water. The disease leads to general lassitude and debility, with serious damage to the kidneys, liver and urinary tract developing in a proportion of cases. There are approximately 200 million people in the world infected with schistosomiasis, of whom 20 million suffer severe consequences. The disease is still found in 74 countries world-wide. Control is complex, but improved water supply helps by reducing contact opportunities with infected waters; a review of epidemiological studies (Esrey et al. 1991) found a median 77 per cent reduction in infection rates through well-designed water and sanitation interventions.

Guinea worm

Dracunculus (the guinea worm) can only be ingested by drinking water that contains the very small crustacean *Cyclops* (the water flea), which acts as an intermediate host. The cyclops breaks down in the stomach, releasing the worm. The female migrates through the body, emerging in a painful blister, usually in the leg, to release eggs into water, from where they return to the cyclops. The principal damage from this disease is temporary disability, both during and after the emergence of the worm; secondary infection occurs in about half of all cases, and disability may last for months.

Guinea worm is the target of an international eradication campaign, and may be the second disease, after smallpox, to be eradicated. Progress has been dramatic over the past ten years, with the number of new cases reported per year dropping by 95 per cent from 890,000 in 1989 to less than 35,000 in 1996 (Periès and Cairncross 1997). The disease is found across Sub-Saharan Africa including Sudan, Nigeria, Ghana, Uganda, and Ethiopia. Chad and Senegal have now declared no new cases and Uganda is close to this point. In South Asia, both Pakistan and India have been certified as 'guinea worm free'.

Water-related vector-borne diseases

These are diseases spread by insects that either breed in water, or are found near water.

Malaria

Malaria is the most significant of these, having a widespread distribution and severe health effects, causing acute and recurring bouts of fever; it is spread by the *Anopheles* mosquito that breeds in still, relatively clean water. The problem is most severe in Africa, southern Asia, South-East Asia, and the South-West Pacific. Central and South America (particularly the Amazon basin) are other problem areas.

- Malaria is responsible for 1.5 to 1.7 million deaths/year, over 90 per cent of these are in Africa.
- There are 300 to 500 million cases of malaria, over 90 per cent of which are in Africa.

Anopheles mosquitoes have a wide variety of possible breeding sites which means that water supplies make relatively little difference to malaria, except in those areas too arid to have any other year-round breeding sites. In such places, water tanks and streams or puddles of spilt water can provide opportunities for

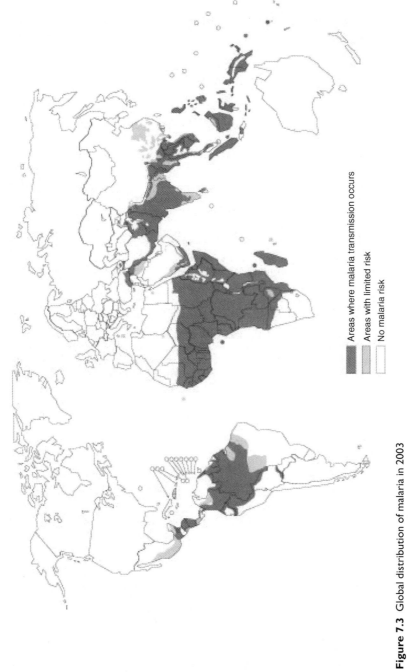

Figure 7.3 Global distribution of malaria in 2003
Source: World Health Organization (2003)

Areas where malaria transmission occurs
Areas with limited risk
No malaria risk

mosquito-breeding throughout the year, creating the risk of falciparam malaria, the more lethal type of the disease.

Filariasis

Filariasis is an infection of parasites spread by urban *Culex* and some rural *Anopheles* mosquitoes, which breed in unsanitary conditions, such as flooded latrines and septic tanks, blocked sewage drains, etc. The parasites may block lymph ducts, leading to the swelling of limbs (elephantiasis) or the scrotum (hydrocele). While many people are infected, the number of clinical cases is far smaller, but can build up to 1 per cent or more in the population over 40 years old.

Dengue

Dengue is a viral infection which leads to acute fevers, and repeated infection can lead to the more serious dengue haemorrhagic fever. Dengue is spread by the domestic day-biting mosquito *Aedes aegypti* which breeds in artificial sources of water, such as that trapped in tin cans and tyres after rainfall, and especially in water storage vessels. Dengue transmission occurs in virtually every low/middle income country (Figure 7.4). As a result, between 50 and 100 million people are infected by the disease. Because dengue cannot be prevented by vaccine or treated with antibiotics, the only available means of control is to prevent mosquito breeding by environmental intervention.

Yellow fever

Yellow fever is another often fatal viral infection transmitted by the same vector as dengue, and consequently having the same links to water and solid waste management as a preventive intervention. It is very much a disease of epidemics; in 1987 over 120,000 cases occurred in the cities of Western Nigeria; in Senegal in 1965, an epidemic was traced to the practice of storing water in containers buried in the ground. Yellow fever is currently restricted to Latin America and Africa.

Onchocerciasis

Onchocerciasis, more commonly known as 'river blindness', is caused by parasites known as microfilariae spread by *Simulium* blackflies which breed in well-aerated rapids. Ironically, it is the *death* of the parasite that can lead to blindness. Disease control consists largely of the use of insecticides and the distribution of the drug invermectin, which kills the parasite *without* consequent damage. The acuteness of the illness varies, so that large numbers of people can be infected without blindness.

Environmental factors in the spread of vector-borne diseases

A number of environmental factors, including the source of the water supply, waste disposal mechanisms and temperature influence the spread of vector-borne diseases. Humidity, vegetation, crop cultivation patterns and housing quality and density are also important. Modification of habitats due to changes in patterns of water use has led to an increase in these diseases. The increasing use of irrigation

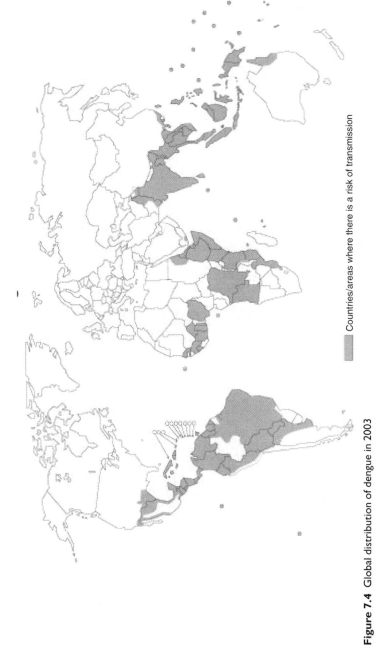

Figure 7.4 Global distribution of dengue in 2003

Source: World Health Organization (2003)

Countries/areas where there is a risk of transmission

Table 7.4 Examples of how changes in environmental conditions increases the spread of vector-borne disease

Disease	Area	Change in environment
Malaria	Amazon	urban development
	Africa, South Asia	poor water management
	SE Asia	deforestation, aforestation, reforestation
	Tropics	increase in irrigation
Schistosomiasis	Sub-Saharan Africa	irrigation schemes and reservoirs
Dengue fever	Urban (some rural) tropical areas	solid waste problems combined with inadequate storage of household drinking water
Filariasis	Urban tropical areas	vectors breed in open sewage canals, blocked drains and waste water used for irrigation
Japanese encephalitis	South and SE Asia	irrigated rice growing areas where cropping patterns have changed

Source: WHO (2004)

and the construction of dams and reservoirs with the related changes in land use have been an important source of vector-borne disease. Poor water management in urban areas has also been implicated. Some of this is the result of the poor planning of projects and lack of communication or cooperation between construction and health sectors in the design of water resources. Table 7.4 outlines some examples of how development can increase the spread of vector-borne disease.

There is a further major environmental influence changing the range of vector-borne diseases – climate change. As the rainfall patterns change and there is a warming of the Earth's surface, the range of vector-borne diseases, particularly malaria, is changing. This is covered in detail later in Chapter 10 where we deal with climate change.

 Activity 7.2

Water-related vector-borne diseases are responsible for millions of lost disability adjusted life years (DALYs) world-wide each year and are an important public health issue in many countries.

What are the main ways that water-related vector-borne disease can be prevented through environmental or other means?

 Feedback

The most effective method of disease reduction is improving water quality and decreasing access to poor supplies. This reduces transmission of water-related disease and also of water-borne, water-washed and water-based diseases. Water-based diseases that are spread through intermediate hosts can be reduced by decreasing the

Table 7.5 Preventing transmission of water-related vector-borne diseases

Disease	Vector	Environmental prevention	Other prevention
Malaria	Anopheles mosquito	Still, relatively clean water – insecticides and other methods to prevent breeding. Draining of water, use of bed nets and insecticides to prevent transmission	Anti-malarial drugs and treatments are available, although there is increasing resistance to some of these substances
Filariasis	Culex and some Anopheles mosquitoes	Vectors breed in unsanitary conditions, such as flooded latrines and septic tanks, blocked sewage drains. Removal of breeding sites through drainage and insecticides	
Dengue	Aedes aegypti mosquito	Artificial water sources – disused cans, tyres, water storage vessels. Removal of breeding sites through drainage and insecticides	No other control method
Yellow fever	Aedes aegypti mosquito	Artificial water sources – disused cans, tyres, water storage vessels. Removal of breeding sites through drainage and insecticides	Vaccination exists
Onchocerciasis	Simulium blackflies	Breed in well-aerated rapids, insecticide is used for control	Invermectin can be taken to kill the parasite without damage

need for contact with the water such as supplying drinking and bathing water through standpipes. Transmission of water-related diseases can additionally be reduced by improving surface water management, thus destroying breeding sites for insects and decreasing the need to visit breeding sites.

Sanitation

To prevent the transmission of disease it is not sufficient merely to supply adequate quantities of clean water. The disposal of waste material from sewerage – sanitation – is also important for maintaining environmental quality and minimizing disease risk. Most ground and surface water pollution in low and middle income countries is due to the discharge of untreated or inadequately treated sewage. In high income countries most sewage is collected by a municipal sewerage system, septic tank or another means. This does not prevent the contamination of the environment as some is pumped out to sea or into rivers or other water sources with little or no treatment. In low and middle income countries, approximately 10 per cent of the population (most of this in urban areas) has access to sewerage systems (WHO 1997).

Human faeces are a risk to human health due to the pathogens they contain. Exposure to these pathogens is usually via contaminated drinking water, food and hands, however, helminthic worms can also enter via the skin. Pathogens associated with human faeces can cause diarrhoea, cholera, intestinal worm infections and typhoid fever. Epidemics are caused when pathogens such as *Vibro cholorae* which causes cholera are introduced into areas with poor sanitation and water supply and poor food safety.

Water pollution (chemical contamination)

Globally, disease transmission associated with the water supply is a substantial health issue, and the most significant global burden of disease related to environmental factors. However, there is increasing public concern about the extent of water pollution due to contamination by chemicals, particularly in high income countries. There is a range of chemical contaminants from a variety of sources, both natural and as the result of human activity.

Table 7.6 Source of chemical constituents of water

Source	Examples
Naturally occurring	Rocks, soils and the effects of the geological setting and climate
Industrial sources and human dwellings	Mining (extractive industries) and manufacturing and processing industries, sewage, solid wastes, urban run-off, fuel leakages
Agricultural activities	Manures, fertilizers, intensive animal practices and pesticides
Water treatment or materials in contact with drinking water	Coagulants, disinfection by-products ('DBPs'), piping materials
Pesticides used in water for public health	Larvicides used in the control of insect vectors of disease
Cyanobacteria	Eutrophic lakes

Quality standards for treated water include setting limits for chemicals and other pollutants that are a hazard to health. It is also important to assess other qualities of the water that may discourage use of that particular source such as an unpleasant taste, odour, appearance or other factor (Cairncross and Feachem 1993). In some areas these other qualities prevent what should be a clean (in bacteriological terms) water supply from being used. Table 7.2 showed some more examples of the way in which water quality is affected by various processes.

There are no standards for untreated water, but efforts should be made to ensure that no chemical pollutants are used that are harmful to health. For instance, Bangladesh has a problem with deep wells that are contaminated with arsenic. This water has physical characteristics that are repellent such as discoloration or odour, and leads to preferential use of surface water sources that are contaminated with bacteria.

Water contaminants

Nutrients and phosphates

Nitrates and phosphates are found in domestic waste water, agricultural run-off and some industrial waste water. These substances are a ready source of nutrients for aquatic organisms and can cause eutrophication of waterways and lakes. This is an increasing problem in different parts of the world. Excess nitrates, particularly from agricultural run-off, are a significant problem and can end up in drinking water, often exceeding the safe levels set by the WHO.

Chemicals in drinking water

There are a number of inorganic and organic compounds that end up in drinking water from natural and man-made sources or as a result of water purification by-products. Many are present in water in very small quantities and have no or unknown health effects. However, some compounds are known to be toxic or carcinogenic if present in drinking water in sufficient concentrations. Other compounds have unpalatable tastes or odours, such as water disinfection with chlorine. Table 7.7 presents a small selection of inorganic chemicals that have health significance in drinking water.

Pesticides

Most exposure to pesticides is via food rather than water and in some circumstances the concentrations are sufficient to be harmful to human health, requiring

Table 7.7 Selection of guideline values for inorganic chemicals that are of health significance in drinking water

Chemical	Guideline value (mg/litre)	Source for guideline
Arsenic	0.01 (P)	Naturally occurring from rocks
Cadmium	0.003	Industrial sources and human dwellings
Cyanide	0.07	Industrial sources and human dwellings
Chromium	0.05 (P)	Naturally occurring from rocks
Fluoride	1.5	The volume of water consumed and intake from other sources should be considered when setting national standards
Mercury	0.001	Industrial sources and human dwellings (total mercury = inorganic plus 'organic')
Selenium	0.01	Naturally occurring
Uranium	0.015 (P, T)	Naturally occurring (only chemical aspects of uranium addressed)

Notes: P = provisional guideline value, as there is evidence of a hazard, but the available information on health effects is limited;
T = provisional guideline value because calculated guideline value is below the level that can be achieved through practical treatment methods, source protection, etc.
Source: WHO (2004)

monitoring. In some parts of the world large amounts of pesticides are applied (herbicides, insecticides, fungicides, molluscicides) and most have tolerable daily allowances determined by the WHO. Where there is run-off from fields to surface water supplies, or where there is treatment of water with insecticides or molluscicides, there is a chance that the pesticide levels will exceed set limits. Detecting the presence of pesticides in water destined for drinking is complex and requires special equipment for analysis. Pesticides in the water supply will also change the local ecology; this is particularly important in those developing countries that use fish caught from surface waters as a significant source of protein in the diet. Some pesticides accumulate in the food chain and can lead to much higher levels of pesticide ingestion in humans than is received through drinking water.

Other organic chemicals such as polycyclic aromatic hydrocarbons (PAHs) are found in water and in some areas, treatment regimes using granular activated carbon are used to reduce the amount of organic chemicals. PAHs are known to cause cancer, but as with pesticides, most exposure is through food and not water.

There are a variety of sources of water pollution, both chemical and biological. Only a few of the chemical sources have been mentioned here; others such as arsenic and fluoride have specific and important health consequences. The protection of water sources from pollution is important to ensure a sufficient and reliable source of acceptable water sources. The cooperation of industry, agriculture, house-holds and local and national authorities is essential to ensure this can happen.

Standard-setting for quality of the water supply

By now you will know about biological and chemical hazards to the supply of clean water and also about the importance of supplying a sufficient quantity of water to all the population. Water quality and treatment standards can only be defined in terms of the purpose for which water is to be used; refer back to Table 7.2 to remind yourself of the various uses for water.

Approaches to standard-setting

In order to provide water of a suitable quality, standards have to be set that define the tolerable level for any contaminants that may be in the water supply. Consider the differences in these three approaches to standard-setting.

1 No acceptable risk: no potentially disease-causing agent should be present in the water.
2 No excess risk: there should be no excess hazard from a contaminant. The dose response relationship is important here. A substance is not a contaminant if we cannot detect an effect. To be on the safe side, the standard will apply a level of the contaminant at a specified fraction below that of a detectable effect. For example, if it is known that 50 organisms/100 cm^3 will make 5 per cent of the population sick, then we will settle for 5 organisms/100 cm^3 and so there is still a finite risk.
3 Economic risk: the best available water, subject to economic constraints and other alternative uses of the money.

Individuals and agencies involved in standard-setting for water quality will take these factors into account when they issue guidelines.

The rest of the chapter is taken up by an activity that looks at some of the issues surrounding quality and standards for water.

Activity 7.3

This activity explores implications of adopting a cost–benefit perspective on standards, as opposed to an absolutist approach of 'safe' or 'unsafe' quality. This raises the potentially controversial notion of differing standards for differing costs or populations, and 'the dollar value of a human life'. The activity will consider different strategies for water pollution management: treatment at pollutant source vs treatment before ingestion.

A water engineer has been asked to select the best options for establishing a rural water supply for a community of 200 people. She has visited the area and after some research is considering using an underground stream that emerges from a nearby hillside as the best source for the water. She is aware that groundwater is usually clean and safe. There is an alternative source available; a large river that also runs close to the village.

She takes some water samples from the underground stream and the large river and sends them to the 'Institut Pasteur' for bacteriological analysis. When the results come back, she presents them in combination with her estimates of the possible quantity of water each source can supply.

After studying the results (Table 7.8), the water engineer is initially considering two options for the supply of safe water to the village; these are set out below.

Table 7.8 Water source, bacteria count and available water

Water source	Bacteria count (E. coli/100 cm^3)	Institut Pasteur verdict	Available water (litres per person per day)
Underground stream	20	Suspected as a contamination source	20
River Styx	1000	Not fit for drinking	200

Option 1: Underground stream

Install a small treatment works which can eliminate all bacteria if properly maintained. Cost: Installation $20(US)/person then $5/person/year cost of chemicals.

Option 2: Large river

Install sedimentation and filtration facilities before chlorination. This is required because occasionally the water is very turbid (muddy) although most of the time it is remarkably clear. Cost: Installation $200(US)/person then $10/person/year cost of chemicals.

The engineer then receives a visit from a local environmentalist who points out that, in addition to pathogenic bacteria, there have been long-standing concerns about upstream pesticide use which may be contaminating the river water. The engineer checks the chemical content of the water for obvious contaminants, and finds 3 μg of DDT (p,p-dichloro-diphenyl-trichloro-ethane) per litre of water, which lies above the recommended water quality guidelines of WHO, which are 2 μg/litre. The engineer is fortunate in that she will be able to remove the DDT from the water for the extra cost of only $20(US)/head.

1 What issues should the engineer consider in order to choose the best option?
2 Should she take the option of removing the DDT from the river water?
3 What other policy options might the state or the pollution control authorities wish to consider?

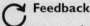

Feedback

1 The first issue to consider is: What is the supply for the community now and what will it require in the future? You will recall that 50 litres per person per day is the minimum necessary water requirement. The problem of using the underground stream, while it has clean water, is that it may not supply a large enough quantity. One possibility may be to use it as the source of drinking water and use the river water for washing and other uses.

The second issue to consider is: Are there any water-related diseases causing a problem in the village already and how can they be best prevented? It may be a sanitation issue – would improved hygiene behaviour be the solution? What are the priorities for those in the village? Will the new water be of better quality than the old water?

The third issue to consider is: What can the community afford to pay and where will the funds come from? How will the supply be maintained and who will pay for it?

2 It will depend partially on how much money is available and whether it is essential to use this water source or whether there are alternate sources. She might need to consider what the DDT standard for her country is.

3 The village will need to consider where the DDT is coming from and how they can control the levels. Is it possible to fine or penalize those who are allowing the DDT to enter the water supply? Are there regulations already and how can limits be enforced?

Summary

Water is a basic human need. The availability of clean water and adequate sanitation facilities varies throughout the world, but it is almost always the poorest communities who are most vulnerable to water-related illness as the technological, financial, or hygiene educational infrastructure may be inadequate. In high income countries water-borne diseases are becoming rarer; with increasing industrialization; chemical water pollution is the main concern. In low and middle income countries by contrast, water-related illnesses are the greater source of ill health and death, although the adverse effects of unregulated industrialization are increasingly taking a toll here as well.

References

Cairncross S, Blumenthal U, Kolsky P, Moraes L and Tayeh A (1996) The public and domestic domains in the transmission of disease. *Tropical Medicine and International Health* 1(1): 27–34.

Cairncross S and Feachem R (1993) *Environmental Health Engineering in the Tropics* (2nd edn). Chichester: John Wiley & Sons, Ltd.

Esrey SA, Potash JB, Roberts L and Shiff C (1991) Effects of improved water supply and sanitation on ascariasis, diarrhoea, dracunculiasis, hookworm infection, schistosomiasis, and trachoma. *Bulletin of the World Health Organization* 69(5): 609–21.

Gleick PH (1996) Basic water requirements for human activities: meeting basic needs. *Water International* 21(2): 83–92.

Gupta A and Asher M (1998) *Environment and the Developing World: Principles, Policies and Management.* Chichester: John Wiley & Sons Ltd.

Kawata K (1978) Water and other environmental interventions: the minimum investment concept. *American Journal of Clinical Nutrition* 31: 2114–23.

Periès H and Cairncross S (1997) Global eradication of Guineau worm. *Parasitology Today* 13: 431–7.

Wagner EG and Lanoix JN (1958) *Excreta Disposal for Rural Areas and Small Communities.* Geneva: WHO.

World Health Organization (1997) *Health and Environment in Sustainable Development.* Geneva: WHO.

World Health Organization (2002) *World Health Report: Reducing Risks, Promoting Healthy Life.* Geneva: WHO.

World Health Organization (2004) *WHO Guidelines for Drinking-Water Quality* (3rd edn). Vol. 1 Recommendations. Geneva: WHO.

Further reading

UN-Habitat (2003) *Water and Sanitation in the World's Cities: Local Action for Global Goals.* London: Earthscan Publications.

Water Aid: http://www.wateraid.org.uk/

World Resources Institute (1998) *World Development Report 1998/9.* Washington, DC: Oxford University Press.

8 | Outdoor air pollution

Overview

Outdoor air pollution is a significant environmental health problem in high, middle and low income countries. You will see in this chapter that there are many sources and types of air pollution, each of which have different health effects. The challenge of air pollution studies – particularly in epidemiology – is to understand how pollutants affect the long- and short-term health of various populations. The information from these studies can then be used to estimate the burden of disease from different sources of air pollution and be an aid to setting standards and managing air quality.

Learning objectives

At the end of this chapter, you will be better able to:

- describe the main components of air pollution of concern to health, and the sources from which they derive
- outline the distinction between the health effects of acute and long-term exposure to air pollution
- discuss standard-setting for air quality
- analyse data from a study on air pollution and mortality, and comment on the uncertainties of the study

Key terms

Particulates Particulate matter, aerosols or fine particles are tiny particles of solid or liquid suspended in the air.

Patient characteristics Characteristics either inherited (e.g. a blood group), or behavioural (e.g. smoking and diet habits) or environmental factors (e.g. exposure to asbestos), associated with an increased or decreased probability (risk) of developing a disease (or other outcome).

Photochemical smog The reaction of hydrocarbons, for example, gasoline or methane, with nitrous oxide gases in sunlight that may lead to reduced visibility.

Primary pollutant A chemical added directly to the atmosphere from natural or human activity.

Secondary pollutant A chemical formed in the atmosphere when primary pollutants react with air, chemicals or sunlight.

Smog A mixture of smoke and fog.

Outdoor air pollution and public health

Air is considered to be polluted when it contains any extraneous constituent in sufficient quantities to adversely affect the environment or the health of people exposed to it. Outdoor air pollution has been the focus of much public and scientific debate in recent years. There is now a growing body of evidence that health effects are linked to pollution even at relatively low concentrations. This translates into a potentially large public health issue in some of the rapidly growing urban areas such as Mexico City, where the provision of public oxygen booths has been proposed to ameliorate the noxious effects of air pollution. Considerable research has now been undertaken to investigate important issues such as the mechanisms responsible, the effects of chronic exposure, how to identify susceptible populations, and the development of management and reduction strategies. Nevertheless, a number of questions remain to be answered. Indoor air pollution will be considered separately in Chapter 9.

Sources of air pollution

Outdoor air pollution originates from a number of different sources, which makes strategies for control difficult. In addition, individual pollutants have different effects on health.

The burning of fossil fuels for energy, and emissions from petrol- and diesel-powered vehicles have been particularly cited as contributing to the poor quality of air in cities. Asthma and other lung diseases, cancer and brain damage are thought to result from the fogs and smogs created by the dense traffic, factories and power stations typical of large industrial cities. Rural areas can also be affected by 'natural' polluting events such as forest fires and volcanic eruptions.

 Activity 8.1

Think about where you live or work: is there noticeable outdoor air pollution? Where does it come from? You might like to return and refine your answers after you have finished reading the chapter.

 Feedback

In the low or middle income countries, the main sources of air pollution are likely to be:

• burning biomass fuel (wood, animal dung and crop residues)

• transport
• fossil fuel-burning power stations

The list is similar for high income countries but there is less burning of biomass fuels and more transport-related and industrial sources of pollution. The balance of sources changes over time as monitoring and control measures come into force. As you will read

later, stricter controls for sulphur dioxide (SO_2) and particulate matter were introduced in Britain in the 1950s, partly as a result of deaths due to an acute pollution
incident.

The principal source of pollutants in most urban areas is road traffic and other
transport-related sources; the exception is sulphur dioxide which originates from
power stations and other industries.

Types of air pollution

Air becomes polluted if the constituents are present in sufficient amounts to affect
the health of humans or animals or to affect vegetation. There are a variety of air
pollutants; those that follow are known as primary pollutants and are responsible
for 90 per cent of all air pollution:

- particles (often referred to as particulate matter – PM)
- sulphur dioxide (SO_2)
- nitrogen oxides (NO_x) including nitrogen dioxide (NO_2)
- carbon monoxide (CO)
- hydrocarbons (CH_x) and photochemical oxidants.

Health effects of the principal types of pollutants

- *Particulates and sulphur dioxide*: Most attention has focused on particle fractions
  (and sulphur dioxide), especially particles of small diameter that can enter the
  respiratory tract. Evidence of adverse health effects is strongest for particles with
  a diameter of less than 10 micrometers (so-called PM10). Those less than 2.5
  micrometers (PM2.5) are respirable, that is small enough to penetrate deep into
  the lung. These last particles are of particular concern as they irritate the lungs
  and may be composed of toxic metals which can be carcinogenic or can cause
  brain, kidney, liver and nerve damage (Stoker and Saeager 1976, in Gupta and
  Asher 1998).
- *Nitrogen oxides (NO_x)*: The health impacts of nitrogen dioxide are not very clear;
  at high levels, NO_2 acts as an irritant and may lead to bronchitis in children.
  Nitrogen monoxide (NO) is released from car engines and is oxidized to NO_2 in
  the atmosphere. The main effect of NO_x gases is their role in the production of
  photochemical smog through their reaction with hydrocarbons.
- *Carbon monoxide (CO)*: Carbon monoxide binds to haemoglobin in the blood
  and can reduce its oxygen-carrying capacity. This is a particular problem for
  people with existing cardio-respiratory limitation.

Other important pollutants are:

- *Ozone (O_3)*: Ozone has been shown to have effects on lung function in some
  subjects, probably through inflammatory or irritant processes.
- *Lead (Pb)*: Lead can bring about behavioural change and brain damage. Most
  lead in the air is 'organic lead' in which it is bonded to a hydrocarbon.

Dispersion and chemistry of pollutants

The effect of a pollutant will depend on the amount and its effectiveness. The relationship between the concentrations of pollutants found in the air and sources of emissions is complex and influenced by patterns of dispersion, air chemistry, and other factors. All emissions undergo chemical or physical transformation to some degree (Figure 8.1).

Low-level ozone and nitrogen dioxide are secondary pollutants formed by chemical reactions of primary pollutants. Although small quantities of NO_2 are emitted by vehicles, most derive from the oxidation of nitrogen oxide (NO) by ozone and the hydroperoxy ($HO_2{}^{\bullet}$) radical:

$$NO + O_3 \rightarrow NO_2 + O_2$$
$$NO^{\bullet} + HO_2{}^{\bullet} \rightarrow NO_2{}^{\bullet} + OH^{\bullet}$$

NO_2 is also the main precursor of ozone in a reaction catalysed by sunlight (hv) and volatile organic compounds:

$$NO_2 \overset{h v}{\rightarrow} NO + O^{\bullet}$$
$$O^* + O_2 \rightarrow O_3 \text{ (where } O^{\bullet} \text{ represents an exited state atom)}$$

High levels of nitrogen dioxide tend to be associated with low levels of ozone and vice versa. Ozone is typically highest in peri-urban and rural areas rather than in city centres, where the NO is thought to react with ozone-forming NO_2.

The type of urban pollution seen in many countries has changed dramatically over the past century with changes in transport and domestic and industrial energy production and use. In the early part of the twentieth century, the main constituent of air pollution in British cities such as London was the emission of sulphur dioxide from burning coal and other fossils fuels; this led to acidic smog.

Since then, with the banning of such fuels in urban areas, concentrations of sulphur dioxide and larger sooty particles have declined dramatically. Now the main problem is photochemical smog from traffic-related emissions, which tend to occur under certain meteorological conditions – notably anti-cyclonic conditions that can lead to a stable layer of air forming above the boundary layer and reducing the movement of air within it, combined with strong sunlight.

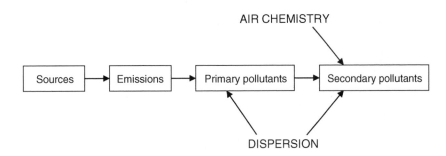

Figure 8.1 Dispersion and air chemistry in relation to pollutants

Activity 8.2

This activity is to remind you of the sources and health effects of air pollution. Use the summary in Table 8.1, together with the information in the first part of the chapter, to answer the following questions:

1 How have most industrialized cities in high income countries managed to clean up their air?
2 What is thought to be the chief type of outdoor air pollutant in low and middle income countries, and what are its sources and effects?
3 How do most air-transmitted pollutants enter the body, and what differences are there in the ways in which the various primary pollutants affect human health?
4 Besides the danger to human health, what other environmental damage is caused by the pollutants described?

Table 8.1 Primary pollutants of outdoor air, principal sources, effects on health and the environment and control methods

Type	Source	Effect on health and environment	Control
Particulates	Industry, biomass combustion, waste incineration, car emissions	Respiratory problems, lung cancer, eye irritation, loss of environmental visibility	Gas cleaning, use less coal and biomass fuels Separate industrial from residential areas Controlled incineration
Sulphur oxides (SO_2 and SO_3)	Biomass and fossil fuel combustion (coal in particular). Industrial emissions	Acid rain damage to vegetation and buildings Corrosion of metals Cardio-respiratory problems	Reduced use, of sulphurous coal Fluidized-bed combustion
Carbon monoxide (CO)	Incomplete combustion in car exhaust and biomass burning. Industry	Nerve and brain dysfunction Cardiac problems, low birthweight, death	Control of vehicle emissions (catalytic converters) Use of public transport
Nitrogen oxides (NO_x)	Transportation, biomass and fossil fuel combustion. Cigarette smoke	Plant damage, photochemical smog, respiratory tract problems	Catalytic converters Reduce traffic volumes; much is secondary reaction
Hydrocarbons and photochemical oxidants, e.g. ozone, aldehydes	Car emissions, industry, incineration Solvent evaporation	Respiratory problems, eye nose and throat irritation Plant damage Photochemical smog	Emission control (catalytic converters) fuel efficiency
Lead	Car emissions (using unleaded petrol)	Behavioural changes and brain damage	Use of unleaded petrol

Feedback

1 Column 4 of Table 8.1 lists control measures used to reduce outdoor air pollution. Many of these have required legislation. You should note that while most of the pollution has resulted from industrialization, rural areas also have problems. There are means of reducing or inhibiting most forms of outdoor air pollution although there are usually economic consequences in controlling them.

2 In rural areas the burning of biomass fuel is the most significant air pollutant; in urban areas, fossil fuel (petrol, diesel, coal) emissions associated with transport and power stations are the most significant.

3 Most air pollutants act on the cardio-respiratory system via the lungs. The effect of particulate matter is a result of size and toxicity. Large particles act as an irritant, causing or exacerbating respiratory symptoms; small particles can carry toxic metals into the lungs, leading to cancer or nerve damage.

4 Particulates can reduce solar radiation and visibility; if they settle on vegetation, they can reduce photosynthesis and damage materials such as textiles and metals. High concentrations of sulphur oxides can damage paints, metals and limestone and marble as well as being responsible for acidic precipitation (see Chapter 11). Ozone and hydrocarbons can damage plants and are involved in the production of photochemical smog.

Studying the health effects of air pollutants

As you have seen, outdoor air pollution has been associated with a number of different health outcomes, including cardiovascular disease, respiratory disease, and cancer. The effect of air pollution on health was shown dramatically in the London smog of December 1952. On this occasion, particulate air pollution reached 1,000 μg/m³. At least 4,000 deaths, mainly cardiovascular, occurred, well in excess of the seasonal average number. This demonstrates the potential acute effects of air pollution; there is also a potential for long-term, chronic effects.

In order to understand the impact of air pollution on health, a variety of study designs are used including:

- laboratory studies on humans and animal models
- population studies: both time series analyses and geographical comparisons.

Laboratory studies use small numbers of subjects, but allow a detailed examination of the physiological and toxicological effects of different pollutants to help establish a mechanism.

Population or epidemiological studies involve larger numbers of people and are concerned with assessing the link between pollutants and health in the general environment. They tend to examine the effects of past exposures to pollution in individual locations over specified periods of time, using time-series analysis. These studies can provide robust evidence of the associations between air pollution and health.

Time-series studies of pollution and mortality links

Daily time-series designs have been used to analyse the associations between acute air pollution and mortality. These studies:

- allow comparison of daily changes in pollution and health
- are methodologically sound, provided the population being analysed remains constant
- require adjustment for time-varying risk factors, including trends, season, day of week, temperature
- provide estimates only of acute effects reflecting exacerbation of disease
- are a key factor in developing causal hypotheses.

Acute health effects

Time-series studies suggest that on days of high pollution, deaths, hospital admissions, and general practice consultations may rise by a few per cent compared with days of low pollution. The APHEA-2 study of 43 million people in 29 European cities found that the estimated increase in daily mortality was 0.6 per cent (95 per cent confidence interval (CI) 0.4 per cent to 0.8 per cent) for each $10 \, \mu g/m^3$ increase in PM10. Cardiovascular deaths increased by 0.69 per cent (95 per cent CI 0.31 per cent to 1.08 per cent) (Katsouyanni et al. 2004). Further analysis of the results suggested that not all of the excess mortality was due to mortality displacement or harvesting. This refers to the excess of deaths during pollution episodes that are probably related to the early deaths of people who already have severe cardio-respiratory disease. In many cases, death may be brought forward only by a day or so; this may deplete the pool of susceptible individuals and the rise in deaths during the episode may, in theory at least, be followed by a compensating decline in cases. If this short-term acceleration of death accounts for all of the excess deaths during a pollution episode, then over the long term, no more deaths would occur than were there to be an absence of air pollution. The deaths are still, however premature. Unfortunately, it is difficult to quantify harvesting effects from time-series analyses.

Similar results have been found in US studies of large populations. The effects are found for cardio-respiratory and all (non-trauma) related mortality; there is also some evidence for increased hospital admission. In studies from a number of different countries, acute particle-based air pollution incidents have been associated with causing cardiac arrhythmias, worsening heart failure, and triggering acute atherosclerotic/ischemic cardiovascular complications (Brook et al. 2004).

Long-term health effects

Chronic or long-term effects may arise through a different mechanism to that for acute effects. It is not possible to quantify chronic effects from daily time-series studies as these specifically remove long-term trends in disease. To study the long-term impact of air pollution, cohort or cross-sectional studies are undertaken to compare the incidence and prevalence of disease in populations exposed to different annual average levels of pollution. They are able to measure years of life lost as well as mortality.

These studies need to take account of the potentially strong confounding effects of economic circumstances, smoking prevalence and other behavioural factors. In common with all population-based studies, there are difficulties in measuring exposure, especially over long periods of time. A recent study analysed time-series and cohort studies and found that time-series analyses can under-estimate cases of death attributable to air pollution and therefore the impact of air pollution on mortality can be better measured by cohort studies (Kunzli et al. 2001).

Does chronic exposure cause disease?

The effects of chronic exposure to air pollution have been the subject of a number of large cohort studies which show that elevated levels of cardiovascular disease are particularly associated with exposure to PM2.5 and sulphates. It has been estimated that people living in the most polluted US cities could lose between 1.8 and 3.1 years of life because of exposure to chronic air pollution (Pope 2000).

What is important is the extent to which new diseases such as more lung cancers or new cases of asthma are induced by chronic exposure over a period of months and years. This is one of the continuing challenges to environmental epidemiology and one for which there remains very little robust evidence.

Most of the outdoor air pollution studies have been carried out in high income countries. It is important that conditions are also studied where there has been huge growth in urban development, particularly in China and India. Knowledge needs to be gained about the types of pollution, the population structure, and the meteorological conditions prevalent in those countries, so that an estimate of the disease burden carried by them can be gained (McMichael and Smith 1999). This is highlighted by the findings of a time-series study in Delhi, India. The authors found a 2.3 per cent rise in non-traumatic deaths per 100 microgram increase in particulates per cubic metre, compared to 6 per cent found elsewhere. The variation in the death rates has been attributed to the differing age structures in the popula-tions (Cropper et al. 1997). Using the data from high income countries on the Delhi population would have overestimated the number of deaths and underestimated the life years saved per death avoided.

Activity 8.3

List some of the barriers to change that policy makers may face when trying to reduce outdoor air pollution.

Feedback

Decisions on public health action are often complicated by other factors such as:

* uncertainty over the clinical importance of air pollution in terms of years of life lost (harvesting)
* reluctance to give up use of private transport
* limited options for alternative energy strategies in growth-based developed economies
* political inertia

Air quality

The nature of urban pollution in Britain and many high income countries has changed dramatically over the past 40 years. Before the UK Clean Air Act of 1956, British cities such as London suffered acidic smogs due to sulphur dioxide emissions from the burning of coal and other fossil fuels.

These atmospheric conditions are still found in many low and middle income countries and in Eastern and Central Europe. China uses sulphurous coal for energy production, industry and home heating. It has been predicted that the number of premature deaths in China due to outdoor air pollution will rise from 200,000 to 500,000 per year by 2020. There is also a high burden of morbidity associated with chronic bronchitis and respiratory illness.

You read earlier about the changing nature of urban air pollution as air quality standards have been introduced and changes take place in energy and transport use. However, some cities in low and middle income countries still have to contend with sulphurous smog-causing pollution from the burning of coal as well as transport-related air pollution.

Setting standards

The ability to maintain and enforce air quality standards necessitates the use of physical, economic and behavioural measures. Examples of physical, economic and behavioural measures that can be used to control air pollution from transportation are:

* physical – lead-free gasoline, catalytic converters; mandatory inspections of emissions
* economic – taxation of ownership; usage and fuel; congestion charges to enter certain areas
* behavioural – use of mass transit systems and alternative travel methods such as walking and cycling; encouraging use of alternative fuels.

Other factors which must be taken into account include the meteorology and topography of the area; the sociodemographic characteristics of the population; the identification of exposed groups; and local and national government participation in air pollution control.

The British example has demonstrated that legislation can be effective in reducing levels of pollutants. Effective legislation, however, requires the development of reliable standards regarding the level of pollutants that can be tolerated without harming public health, and what constitutes 'clean air'. Standards are set by different agencies in different countries, and their principal role is to protect public health.

Air quality, concepts and standards

Air quality standards are set to ensure that pollutants are below harmful levels for humans, animals, vegetation or materials. There are three main types of standards:

- measurement of ambient air quality, with concentrations of major pollutants measured separately
- overall quality of the air
- emission limits for industrial plants.

There are often primary standards which set emission limits to protect public health with an adequate margin of safety, and secondary standards that are set at an even higher level. The standards are set by legislation in different countries or regions and are at different levels; for example, the European Union has developed guidelines for all of Europe and these are now being taken up outside of the original intended geographical area. These standards are based on expert advice. There is extensive documentation to support the guidelines and allow legislators to set the standards in law. The standards will vary between and within countries as each interprets the evidence and analyses the costs and benefits of setting standards at particular levels. This is clearly illustrated in Table 8.2, showing the standards used by Saudi Arabia, the UK, India and WHO.

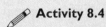 **Activity 8.4**

Look closely at the standards set out in Table 8.2. What are the similarities and differences between the various standards?

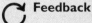 **Feedback**

- Note that not all countries use the same average time for setting standards, for example, 1-, 8- and 24-hour limits are all used.
- In the case of particulate matter, different sizes (micrometers) are measured.
- There are also differing thresholds set for exceeding the guidelines.
- Even when the same hourly average is used, the standards differ.
- Countries have identified different pollutants as priorities for standard-setting, e.g. all have included lead and particulate matter, but only Saudi Arabia has included ammonia.
- The availability of suitable technology and differences in political will has an influence upon the final setting of standards.

Table 8.2 Air pollution standards in a selection of countries and WHO

Pollutant	Averaging	Saudi Arabia[1] μg/m³ (ppm)	UK[2] μg/m³	India[3] μg/m³	India[3] μg/m³	WHO[4] μg/m³	WHO[4] μg/m³
Sulphur	15 minute	730					
	1-hour						
	24-hours	365 (0.140)*					100–150*
	Yearly	80 (0.030)					40–60
Particulate Inhalable	24-hours	340*					
	Yearly	80	50				
Suspended	Annual			360	140	70	60–90
	24-hours			500	200	100	150–230*
Respirable	Annual			120	60	50	
	24-hours			150	100	75	
Ozone (O₃)	1-hour	295					
	8 hour mean		100 (50)				
Oxides of nitrogen (NOₓ)	1-hour	660		80	60		
	Yearly	100 (0.050)				15	
	24-hours			120	80	30	150
Carbon monoxide (CO)	1-hour	40000		10.0	4.0	2.0	40*
	8-hours	10000 (9)**	11.6 (10)	5000.0	2000.0	1000.0	10*

Pollutant	Averaging period						
Hydrogen sulphide (H₂S)	1-hour	200 (0.140)*					
	24-hours	40 (0.030)*					
Ammonia	1-hour	1800 (2.60)*					
Non-methane	3-hours	160 (0.24)					
Lead (Pb)	3-month annual mean	1.5	0.25	1	0.75	0.5	
	24-hours			1.5	1	0.75	
Benzene 1,3-	running	5ppb					
	running	1ppb					0.5–1

Notes: * exceeded no more than once a year

** exceeded no more than twice in a 30 day period

1. Presidency of Meteorology and Environment, http://www.pme.gov.sa/AirQS.asp (2004)
2. The Air Quality Strategy for England, Scotland, Wales and Northern Ireland. Department for the Environment, Food and Rural Affairs in partnership with the Scottish Executive, The National Assembly for Wales and the Department of the Environment for Northern Ireland (2000).
3. National Ambient Air quality Standards (NAAQS) http://dpcc.delhigovt.nic.in/airstd.htm (2004)
4. WHO standards 1992 (in Gupta and Asher, 1998: 165)

Management of air quality in low and middle income countries

The management of air quality requires a multidisciplinary approach which involves government and regulatory bodies as well as industry and individuals. There are legislative powers available to governments as well as technical approaches to control emissions at source. One of the concerns for low and middle income countries is that as the economy grows and more energy is used, air pollution will increase. For example, the economy of China has developed rapidly in the past two decades. Economic activity is associated with an increase in energy consumption and therefore an increase in emissions, leading to a worsening air quality. Coal remains the main source of energy.

China has introduced a number of control measures for air pollution and, as a result, the ambient air quality in a number of large cities in China has actually improved. The source of air pollution in the cities has changed from being primarily coal combustion, to being a mix of combustion and motor vehicle emissions. This has meant that the levels of total suspended particulates and SO_2 in ambient air have decreased in the past 10 years. Conversely, the increasing number of motor vehicles has meant an increase in the ambient air NO_x. There have been a number of studies on the health effects from air pollution in China and they have revealed both acute and chronic effects on mortality, morbidity, hospital admissions, clinical symptoms and lung function changes (Chen et al. 2004).

Estimating the burden of disease resulting from air pollution

A step-by-step guide will now be provided to illustrate how you might estimate the effect of exposure to outdoor air pollution on mortality. The guide is based on a study carried out in London by Anderson and colleagues (1996), which measured air pollution levels and daily mortality between 1987 and 1992. This study was chosen because it is a good example of time-series analysis and the principles involved in this study could be applied elsewhere.

Air pollution and daily mortality in London, 1987–1992

- *Objective*: To investigate whether outdoor air pollution levels in London influence daily mortality.
- *Design*: Time-series regression analysis of daily counts of deaths, with adjustment for effects of secular trend, seasonal and other cyclical factors, day of the week, holidays, influenza epidemic, temperature, humidity, and autocorrelation, from April 1987 to March 1992. Pollution variables were particles black smoke (a measure of particles in the air), sulphur dioxide, ozone and nitrogen dioxide, lagged 0–3 days.
- *Setting*: Greater London.
- *Outcome measures*: Relative risk of death from all causes (excluding accidents), respiratory disease, and cardiovascular disease.
- *Results*: Black smoke concentrations on the previous day were significantly associated with all causes of mortality, and this effect was also greater in the warm season, independent of the effects of other pollutants. An increase in black smoke from 8 to 22 $\mu g/m^3$ was associated with a 1.7 per cent increase in daily mortality from all causes. The median (the middle of a distribution of numbers (50th percentile)) concentration

of black smoke over this period was 13 μg/m³. The median number of deaths in London was 172 per day. A similar association was found for ozone, but smaller and less consistent effects were observed for nitrogen dioxide and sulphur dioxide.
- *Conclusion*: Daily variations in air pollution within the range currently occurring in London may have an adverse effect on daily mortality.

To estimate the total number of deaths likely to be caused by particulate air pollution in London (the total burden of deaths), you will have to make an important assumption: that there is a causal association between black smoke and mortality. The steps to be taken to determine numbers of avoidable deaths are listed below:

1 *Calculation of the percentage of deaths.* Deaths associated with air pollution are expressed in terms of the percentage increase in mortality for each μg/m³ increase in the concentration of black smoke. Assuming that there is a linear relation between mortality and black smoke, you know that the percentage increase in deaths following an increase in black smoke concentration from 8 to 22 μg/m³ (= 14 μg/m³) was 1.7 per cent. This means that the increase in daily deaths per μg/m³ of black smoke is

$$1.7 / 14 = 0.121\%$$

2 *Calculation of the number of deaths.* To understand the public health implications of black smoke, you would want to know the actual number of deaths involved. Use the median number of deaths per day (172). The average increase in daily deaths per μg/m³ of black smoke is thus

$$172 \times 0.121 / 100 = 0.208$$

3 *Calculation of number of avoidable deaths per day.* To understand the relationship between mortality and exposure better, you would want to calculate how many deaths you could avoid if there were no particulate air pollution.

   You can simulate this by extending the linear relationship between mortality and black smoke down to a concentration of 0 μg/m³. You will now be able to estimate the average number of deaths per day that would have been avoided if there had been no particulate air pollution on a day:

   Number of extra deaths per μg/m³ of black smoke = 0.208 × the actual concentration of black smoke = number of deaths avoided if the concentration had been 0.

Note that the average of deaths avoided at 12 and 14 μg/m³ is equal to that avoided at 13 μg/m³.

   You can also calculate the average number of deaths avoided on days with concentrations of black smoke of:
   (a)   13 μg/m³: 0.208 × 13 = 2.70 deaths avoided.
   (b)   12 μg/m³: 0.208 × 12 = 2.50 deaths avoided.
   (c)   14 μg/m³: 0.208 × 14 = 2.91 deaths avoided.
   Average: (2.50 + 2.91) / 2 = 2.70.

4 *Calculation of number of avoidable deaths per year.* If the daily concentrations of black smoke have a symmetrical (even) distribution, then over the course of a year, exposures greater than the median (more than 13 μg/m³) will be matched by exposures less than 13 μg/m³. We can use this information about the distribution of exposure to calculate the average number of daily deaths which could be avoided over one year if there was no exposure to black smoke. If the exposure were reduced to 0 μg/m³ the number of deaths avoided would equal the number

avoided on a day of 13 µg/m³. Using this argument we can calculate the number of deaths that would be avoided over one year if there was no exposure to black smoke:

> Days in a year (365) deaths avoidable at 13 µg/m³ (2.70) = deaths avoidable/ year. 365 × 2.70 = 986 deaths could be avoided in one year if there was no black smoke exposure.

5 *Calculation of percentage of avoidable deaths.* The number of deaths avoided per year should now be changed to a percentage of the total number of deaths:

> Total deaths expected in one year 365 × 172 = 62 780.
> Deaths due to black smoke = 986.
> Deaths due to black smoke / total of all deaths (986 / 62 780) = 1.6%.

This means that in one year 1.6 per cent of the deaths are the result of exposure to black smoke.

6 The main assumptions about the data include the following.
   (a) The relationship between black smoke and death is causal, i.e., black smoke causes extra deaths.
   (b) The relationship between amount of exposure and number of deaths is linear – you assumed that the relationship was a straight line, but the dose–response curve could be a number of shapes.
   (c) Particulate air pollution is adequately indicated by measured black smoke – that black smoke measures the aetiologically important fraction of particulate pollution.
   (d) The slope of the linear relationship is 1.7 per cent.
   (e) The distribution of daily black concentrations is symmetrical – there could be a large number of days when the exposure is quite low, and just a few when it is very high.
   (f) When we state 'deaths caused by air pollution', we include deaths that may have been brought forward by only a short time, possibly only a few days.

 Activity 8.5

If you were explaining the risks of air pollution from black smoke based on this example, what information would you wish to provide when communicating to:

1 an expert committee considering standards for particulate air pollution
2 the general public?

 Feedback

1 (a) You would want to elaborate the measures of uncertainty in your calculations. You could start with using the confidence limits of the slope, but ideally, uncertainty should be reflected in each of the assumptions above.

   (b) Include estimates of the relationship between black smoke and daily death that have been calculated for other places, or by using other assumptions.

2 To present this information to the public, you would want to give them a simplified version of the information you provided to the experts. You could also include some estimates of risk from other exposures or behaviours (such as risk due to traffic accidents, occupational exposures, smoking, and radon exposure). By showing other

risks (a comparative risk analysis), you would enable the reader to put the significance of black smoke exposure in context.

Summary

This chapter has covered the main sources and health effects of outdoor air pollution. Different methods for estimating the potential burden of disease from air pollution were discussed. Time-series analysis and cohort studies were covered in more detail, and a step-by-step guide covered the analysis and uncertainties of a specific air pollution episode. Research evidence demonstrates that both acute and chronic effects of air pollution lead to increased rates of mortality and morbidity. The effects of outdoor air pollution are likely to be different in low and middle income countries. Standard-setting and public health concerns were also discussed.

References

Anderson HR, de Leon AP, Bland JM, Bower JS and Strachan DP (1996) Air pollution and daily mortality in London: 1987–92. *British Medical Journal* 312: 665–9.

Brook RD, Franklin B, Cascio W et al. (2004) Air pollution and cardiovascular disease: a statement for healthcare professionals from the Expert Panel on Population and Prevention Science of the American Heart Association. *Circulation* 109: 2655–71.

Chen B, Hong C and Kan H (2004) Exposures and health outcomes from outdoor air pollutants in China. *Toxicology* 198(1–3): 291–300.

Cropper ML, Simon NB, Alberini A and Sharma PK (1997) The Health Effects of Air Pollution in Delhi, India. World Bank Policy Research Working Paper #1860: http://www-.worldbank.org/nipr/work_paper/1860/netcen

Gupta A and Asher M (1998) *Environment and the Developing World: Principles, Policies and Management.* Chichester: John Wiley & Sons Ltd.

Katsouyanni K, Touloumi G, Samoli E et al. (2001) Confounding and effect modification in the short-term effects of ambient particles on total mortality: results from 29 European cities within the APHEA2 Project. *Epidemiology* 12: 521–31.

Kunzli N, Medina S, Kaiser R, Quenel P, Horak F Jr and Studnicka M (2001) Assessment of deaths attributable to air pollution: should we use risk estimates based on time series or on cohort studies? *American Journal of Epidemiology* 153(11): 1050–5.

McMichael AJ and Smith KR (1999) Seeking a global perspective on air pollution and health. *Epidemiology* 10(1): 1–4.

Pope CA (2000) Epidemiology of fine particulate air pollution and human health: biologic mechanisms and who's at risk? *Environmental Health Perspectives* 108: 713–23.

Pope CA, Burnett RT, Thurston GD et al. (2004) Cardiovascular mortality and long-term exposure to particulate air pollution: epidemiological evidence of general pathophysiological pathways of disease. *Circulation* 109: 71–7.

Royal Commission on Environmental Pollution (1994) 18th report, *Transport and the Environment*, 23. London: HMSO.

Further reading

McGranahan G and Murray F (2003) *Air Pollution and Health in Rapidly Developing Countries.* London: Earthscan.

9 The indoor environment

Overview

The quality of the environment inside our houses, schools and workplaces is important for maintaining good health. The quality of the indoor environment is affected by how we cook and prepare food indoors; how our home and workplaces are built; how services are provided; how they are heated and whether they are overcrowded. This chapter gives an overview of all these aspects and concentrates on the importance of indoor air pollution in low and middle income countries.

Learning objectives

By the end of this chapter, you will be better able to:

- give examples of some of the traditional and modern hazards associated with the indoor environment
- explain the health hazards of indoor pollution, especially for women and children
- describe the importance of indoor temperatures for the prevention of excess winter mortality
- explain the difficulties in estimating the burden of disease from indoor air pollution

Key terms

Attributable risk function The proportion of disease among the exposed that is attributable to the exposure.

Biomass fuel Animal dung, wood or crop residues.

The relationship between the indoor environment and health

As we spend so much time indoors rather than outside (Figure 9.1), the maintenance of a good quality indoor environment is essential for good health. This chapter is concerned with the overall quality of the indoor environment, particularly in the home. The quality of the indoor environment in occupational settings such as schools and the workplace is also very important, but is not the primary focus in this chapter. The indoor environment should also be seen in relation to the outdoor environment because services are provided from outside the home, air

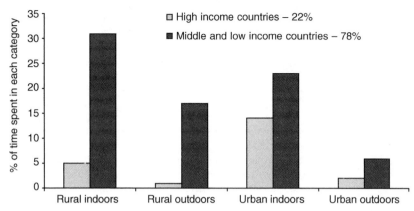

Figure 9.1 Time spent indoors and outdoors by population
Source: Schwela (1996)

pollution and wastes are removed from the home and housing is situated within a physical and social community.

Hazards of the indoor environment

The indoor domestic environment varies widely both within and between countries. The distinction between traditional and modern hazards is marked in the indoor environment; even when homes have 'modern' hazards to contend with, the importance of traditional hazards is not reduced in their public health impact.

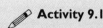 **Activity 9.1**

You were introduced to the concept of traditional and modern hazards in Chapter 3; in this activity you will define them in relation to the indoor environment. To remind you of the definitions, traditional hazards are those that people have been exposed to in the agricultural and early stages of industrial development, whereas modern hazards are mostly of the twentieth and twenty-first century and are associated with high population density and technological innovation:

1 Make a list of traditional and modern hazards associated with an indoor environment and housing.
2 Think of how these hazards influence health.

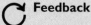 **Feedback**

1 Table 9.1 gives examples of just a few of the hazards you might have thought of.

Table 9.1 Traditional and modern hazards associated with the indoor environment

Traditional hazards	Modern hazards
indoor air pollution from biomass fuels	indoor air pollution from tobacco smoke, asbestos, etc.
inadequate sanitation	cleaning solutions
overcrowding	use of gas appliances
	chemicals used in furnishings etc.

2 Homes in countries at different stages of development will experience different indoor environmental hazards as they transfer predominately traditional to modern hazards. Table 9.2 summarizes a variety of hazards, and their association via population health. A mix of hazards will lead to an increased burden on the population.

Table 9.2 Hazards of the indoor environment and populations at risk

Setting	Hazard	Population at risk	Outcome
High income countries	radon-exposure	those who live or work there	lung cancer
	office and commercial buildings	workers	'sick building syndrome' Asthma
	private residences	general population	solvent-related symptoms; legionnaires' disease; other infections
Low and middle income countries	homes where biomass fuel used for cooking and heating	women and children	acute respiratory infection; chronic obstructive lung diseases; lung cancer

Aspects of housing and health

Building design, building materials and construction-related problems

Accidents in the home are one of the leading causes of injury world-wide. When houses are over-crowded and built of poor quality materials, the incidence of accidents increases significantly. The type of dwelling, and how it is constructed, are important determinants of health in the indoor environment. If building standards are ineffective or non-existent, as in a slum development, there are risks of fire, explosion, collapse, accidents and pollution. For example, poorly designed buildings and fittings can lead to falls, particularly by the elderly and young children. If shelters are made of flammable materials, or cooking fires and stoves are unsafe, the risk of death and injury due to fire are increased. Finally, poor design in the layout of the room can lead to inadequate space and ventilation for cooking, and problems with hygiene. The appropriate design and construction of buildings can help to mitigate the impact of disasters such as earthquakes and hurricanes. This is discussed further in Chapter 12.

High-rise buildings, especially where building standards are poor, carry the risk of fire, explosion or collapse. This can affect large numbers of people. There are often problems maintaining equipment, and vandalism can be rife, particularly in poor areas. High-rise buildings have also been shown to have a negative effect on mental health and to increase the social isolation of inhabitants.

Building materials themselves may be harmful; asbestos was formerly widely used, chiefly as a fire retardant, in commercial and domestic buildings as well as schools and hospitals. It has now been shown to be a toxic material that causes lung cancer and mesothelioma. The resulting cost of removing this from buildings or dealing with it after demolition is enormous. Other building materials such as urea foam insulation and MDF (medium density fibreboard) contain formaldehyde which has been linked to respiratory irritation.

Radon is released from granite and other igneous rocks and has been associated with lung cancer in some studies; if dwellings are built in areas where high levels of radon are present, they need to be designed to reduce exposure to the inhabitants.

Finally, the conditions of the indoor environment are also influenced by the location of the dwelling (i.e. urban, industrial or rural) and the provision of amenities.

Hazards of housing

Table 9.3 summarizes the health outcomes associated with some housing-related hazards. Table 9.3 was designed to catalogue hazards typically found in a home,

Table 9.3 Range of housing-related hazards and associated health outcomes

Housing-related hazard	Health outcome
Asbestos	mesothelioma; lung cancer; pleural plaques
Carbon monoxide	death; neuro-psychological impairment
Cold	cardio-respiratory disease; winter death; respiratory ailments
Damp and mould	rhinitis; asthma; respiratory disease
Domestic hygiene	anaphylactic shock; allergy; asthma
Food safety	food poisoning; diarrhoea; vomiting
Personal hygiene	diarrhoea
Heat	cardiovascular death; myocardial infarction; stroke
Lead	lead poisoning; impaired intelligence
Noise	psycho-physiological effects; hypertension; sleep disturbance; reduced performance
VOCs and biocides	eye disorders; asthma
Other gaseous combustion	cardio-respiratory illness; asthma; sick building syndrome
MMMF	lung cancer; non-malignant respiratory disease; contact dermatitis
Radon	lung cancer
Sanitation	gastro-enteritis
Water	diarrhoea; cryptosporidiosis; legionnaires' disease
Fire	lung damage, burns, death
Falls	fractures, head injury, death

and was used to establish standards of housing safety. The items there illustrate that the harms associated with each hazard range from death to minor illness or injury. Collation of all the hazards permits an overall picture of the quality of the housing stock. This reflects the reality of living in a house with many potential hazards, and allows one to think about measures to alleviate the harm by reducing specific hazards (DETR 2003).

Over-crowding

Over-crowding is a traditional hazard present in high, middle and low income countries. Over-crowding sometimes occurs as a result of traditional multi-generational family units living together in houses designed for smaller families. Generally, over-crowding is associated with poverty and is the result of necessity rather than choice. Individuals may each have less than $1m^3$ of space in some homes. When conditions become crowded there is increased risk of transmission of diseases such as influenza, meningitis, diarrhoea and tuberculosis (Howden-Chapman 2002). Diet in these households is often poor, and malnutrition can increase the susceptibility of inhabitants to diseases of over-crowding. Over-crowding is also associated with violence and with psycho-social disorders. The effects of psychological stress are important, particularly for women who often spend more time in the home than men. Children are also particularly vulnerable to the diseases and the stresses of over-crowding because of the time they spend in the home, and having little room to play or study can negatively impact on their development.

Cold housing and excess winter mortality

Another aspect of the indoor environment is temperature. Excess cold or heat is associated with an increase in mortality and morbidity due to cardio-respiratory illness. Individuals are exposed to health hazards if they are unable to compensate for changes in temperature due to design or inadequate heating or cooling systems in their houses.

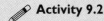 Activity 9.2

Read the extract on cold houses and health from Wilkinson and colleagues (2001). While you are reading, think about how you would target interventions to prevent cold-related winter excess mortality, to maximize the improvement in public health.

Cold houses and health

Britain, despite having relatively mild winters has a large winter excess of death, which results in 40,000 more deaths during December to March than would be expected from the death rates in other months of the year. Some of the excess can be attributed to influenza, respiratory infections, lack of sunlight, diet, and other seasonal factors, however, 60 per cent is associated with the effects of cold. The winter excess is greater than in most other countries of continental Europe and Scandinavia which experience much colder winter conditions. It has been suggested that some of the explanation for this may lie in the quality of the housing stock in Britain, which is less thermally efficient than that in most other North European countries and hence may afford less protection against the cold. To try and better understand the effect of cold on excess winter mortality a study published in 2001 (Wilkinson et al. 2001) looked at the effect of housing stock and thermal efficiency in England and found that:

- There was a 23 per cent excess of deaths from heart attacks and strokes during winter (December to March) compared with non-winter months, much of this can be attributed to cold. Mortality rose by around 2 per cent for each degree Celsius fall in outdoor temperature below 19° Celsius.
- The winter rise in deaths was greatest in older people, but there was some increase for all age groups.
- The risk of excess winter death showed little variation with socioeconomic group.
- The magnitude of the winter excess was greater in people living in dwellings that appear to be poorly heated. The percentage rise in deaths in winter was greater in those dwellings with low energy-efficiency ratings, and those predicted to have low indoor temperatures during cold periods.
- There was a gradient of risk with age of the property, the risk being greatest in dwellings built before 1850, and lowest in the more energy-efficient dwellings built after 1980.
- Private rented dwellings and those that are owner-occupied have more excess deaths, many of the local authority and housing association houses are more modern.
- Damp houses are also a risk factor for excess mortality.
- Absence of central heating and dissatisfaction with the heating system also showed some association with increased risk of excess winter death.
- The indoor temperature in many dwellings appears to fall below 16° Celsius during cold periods. The minimum temperature recommended in the UK to maintain health is 18° C in the living room (16° C in other rooms) and the standard temperature to achieve comfort is 21° C in the living rooms and 18° C elsewhere. Low indoor temperatures were found to be more likely if the dwelling was old, had no or inadequate central heating, was costly to heat, or was occupied by a household with low income. Those who live in local authority or housing association dwellings appeared to be especially likely to have low indoor temperatures during cold periods if their heating costs were high. The disadvantage of having a difficult-to-heat home appeared to be greater in households with low income.

The increase in mortality with cold was greater in homes predicted to have comparatively low indoor temperatures, though the variation between the warmest and coldest houses was fairly small. The marked seasonal fluctuation in mortality was considerably larger in poorly heated homes compared with that in well-heated homes. This is shown in more detail in Figure 9.2.

The findings suggest that indoor temperature and factors associated with poor thermal efficiency of dwellings, including property age, are associated with increased vulnerability to winter death from diseases of the heart and circulation. This suggests that substantial public health benefits can be expected from measures that improve the thermal efficiency of dwellings and the affordability of heating them.

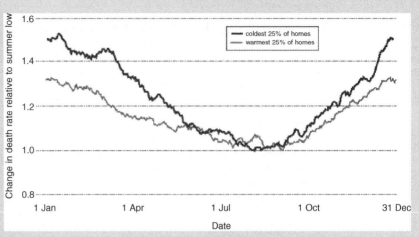

Figure 9.2 Seasonal fluctuation in mortality in cold and warm homes
Source: Wilkinson et al. (2001)

↻ **Feedback**

To decrease the number of winter deaths, any intervention has to target the population most likely to benefit. The most vulnerable groups are the elderly living in old damp houses, and those which are private rented or owner-occupied. Therefore, improving the energy efficiency of houses by improving insulation and installing or upgrading heating systems should reduce excess winter mortality if it results in an increase in internal temperature and a reduction in dampness. It is not just living in energy-inefficient housing that is the cause of low internal temperatures; fuel poverty (having to spend more than 10 per cent of household income on fuel) is another problem in the UK. There is now an annual winter fuel payment for pensioners aimed at allowing those on low incomes to better heat their houses without having to forgo other essentials of daily living. The government developed a Home Energy Efficiency Scheme to try to improve the housing stock, targeted in the first instance at the elderly and those on low incomes. An evaluation has been carried out to ascertain whether the correct groups were being targeted and are taking advantage of the improvements offered by this scheme. The evaluation aimed to measure the changes in temperature and dampness due to the interventions and to quantify the health benefits (both physical and psycho-logical) from improvements in housing. This has yet to be published, but work carried out in New Zealand (Howden-Chapman et al. 2000) suggests that the psychological benefits of having a warm house are important and that improvements to housing stock are not only a benefit to physical well-being.

Damp housing

The presence of damp and subsequent mould growth in the home has been consistently linked to a number of health outcomes in studies in high income countries. These include nausea, vomiting and respiratory illness. Housing that is damp and prone to condensation tends to be poorly maintained and is associated with the socioeconomic deprivation of the householder. To understand the independent effects of damp on health, it has to be separated from the other effects of poor housing and ill health.

Humidity in the dwelling can cause condensation which encourages the development of fungal spores. Damp is also associated with an increase in house dust mites. Both of these are known allergens, suggesting a causal link with respiratory disease, in particular asthma, and exposure to damp and mould (Peat et al. 1998). In addition there is an observed dose–response relationship, with asthma severity increasing with increasing levels of damp and mould in the home. Keeping a dwelling between 40 and 60 per cent humidity and improving ventilation decreases the numbers of mites that can cause illness.

Principles of healthy housing

The impact of the indoor environment on health in all parts of the world has been introduced in this chapter. Table 9.4 lists some principles of healthy housing published by the WHO in 1989 and is still relevant today. Table 9.4 illustrates how both the physical and social environment of homes can influence the health

Table 9.4 Principles of healthy housing

Protection against communicable disease through:
- safe water supply
- sanitary disposal of excrement
- disposal of other solid wastes
- drainage of surface water
- personal and domestic hygiene
- safe food preparation
- structural safeguards

Protection against injuries, poisonings and chronic diseases through attention to:
- structural features and furnishings
- indoor air pollution
- chemical safety
- use of the home as workplace

Reduction of psychological and social stress through:
- adequate living space, privacy and comfort
- personal and family security
- access to recreation and community amenities
- protection against noise

Access to a supportive living environment through provision of:
- security and emergency services
- health and social services
- access to cultural and other amenities

Protection of populations at special risk
- women and children
- displaced and mobile populations
- the aged, ill and disabled

Source: Adapted from WHO (1989)

of the occupants. The principles governing the promotion of healthy housing are concerned with alleviating both modern and traditional hazards. For example, the spread of communicable disease can be reduced by providing a safe water supply and the likelihood of poisoning can be reduced by attention to chemical safety.

Indoor air pollution in low and middle income countries

The World Bank has identified indoor air pollution in low and middle income countries as one of the most important environmental global concerns today. Globally, people in high income countries spend just 2 per cent of their time in the urban outdoors, however, until recently, most air pollution studies and mitigation efforts have been focused on outdoor pollution in low income countries. The quality of the indoor air is more significant for a much larger portion of the world population, including people in low and middle income countries who spend 54 per cent of their time indoors in both rural and urban settings (World Bank 1993).

About half of the world's population use biomass or solid fuels to provide energy for cooking and heating. These are a major source of indoor particulate concentrations. Table 9.5 describes the loss of Disability adjusted life years (DALYs) that can be attributed to the use of solid fuels. Women in all parts of the world have the greatest burden from indoor smoke because they tend to be in charge of the cooking. Women in low and middle income countries such as Bangladesh, Ecuador and Somalia have the highest attributable risk fraction.

Women and children are the groups most likely to be in close proximity to this source of pollution, due to the time that they spend indoors. These groups are directly engaged in activities which cause indoor pollution such as cleaning and cooking. Respiratory infections account for around 9 per cent of the total global burden of disease for morbidity and mortality, and children under 5 in developing countries account for 80 per cent of that total; a serious public health issue.

Table 9.5 Selected population attributable risk fractions for indoor smoke from solid fuels, by sex and level of development (% Disability Affected Life Years (DALYs))

	World (%)	World (%)	World (%)	Developing country – high mortality (%)		Developing country – low mortality (%)		Developed country (%)	
	Male	Female	ALL	Male	Female	Male	Female	Male	Female
Chronic obstructive pulmonary disease	13	34	22	13	45	16	40	1	4
Lower respiratory infections	36	36	36	41	41	20	21	10	11

Source: WHO (2000)

Indoor air pollution by source

Indoor air pollution is not only as a result of biomass fuel combustion. The indoor environment can be polluted from sources originating outdoors as well as those from inside. Table 9.6 lists a variety of indoor air pollutants by source. Pollution from outside sources such as traffic and industry contributes to indoor as well as outdoor pollution levels. The quality of the design and build of the dwelling determine how well the property is ventilated. Ventilation allows gas, fuel burning and organic solvents, and other agents to dissipate, and also allows the outdoor air in. Personal behaviour influences exposures to indoor air pollutants, for example, using cleaning materials, opening windows, cooking methods and using heating appliances and smoking.

Biomass fuels

Biomass fuels account for 25 per cent of energy provision in low and middle income countries. Open fires for cooking and heating are common in rural and

Table 9.6 Principal air pollutants for indoor environments

Principal pollutants	Sources: predominately outdoor
SO_2, SPM/RSP	fuel combustion, smelters
O_3	photochemical reactions
pollens	trees, grass, weeds, plants
lead (Pb), manganese (Mn)	automobiles
lead, cadmium (Cd)	industrial emissions
VOC's (volatile organic compounds), PAH (polycyclic aromatic hydrocarbons)	petrochemical solvents, vaporization of unburned fuels
	indoor and outdoor
No_x, CO	fuel burning
CO_2	fuel burning, metabolic activity
SPM/RSP	ETS, re-suspension of dust, condensation of vapours and combustion products
water vapour	biological activity, combustion, evaporation
VOC's	volatilization, fuel burning, paint, pesticides, etc.
spores	fungi, moulds
	predominately indoor
radon	soil, building construction materials, water
HCHO	insulation, furnishing, ETS
asbestos	fire retardant insulation
ammonia (NH_3)	cleaning products
polycyclic hydrocarbons, arsenic, nicotine, acrolien VOC	ETS
Mercury (Hg)	adhesives, solvents, cooking, cosmetics
aerosols	fungicides, paints, spills
allergens	consumer products, house dust
pathogenic organisms	house dust, animal dander infections

Source: Adapted from WHO (1995)

peri-urban areas of low and middle income countries. The fire is usually at floor level, often with a tripod or bricks on which to rest cooking pots; this design can result in accidents and problems with food hygiene. There is often no chimney to remove smoke and, as biomass fuels often burn inefficiently, there are high levels of particulates and pollutants in comparison with other fuel sources. Burning of solid fossil fuels such as coal can lead to similar problems, particularly if the fuel is of poor quality and burns inefficiently. The indoor concentration of health-damaging pollutants from a typical wood-fired cooking stove creates carbon monoxide and other noxious fumes at anywhere between seven and five hundred times the allowable limits, far exceeding international safety standards, shown in Table 9.7.

Table 9.7 Pollutant levels from wood-burning stoves

Pollutant	Emission (mg/m³)	Allowable standard (mg/m³)
Carbon monoxide	150	10
Particles	3.3	0.1
Benzene	0.8	0.002
1,3-Butadiene	0.002	0.0003
Formaldehyde	0.7	0.1

Note: Pollutants emitted using 1 kg of wood/hour in 15 ACH 40 m³ kitchen.
Source: Based on UNDP/DESA/WEC (2004)

Rural women and their families also pay a high economic price when collecting biomass fuels. Time spent looking for wood could be spent on more productive paid work, raising the family income and helping to improve the standard of living and nutritional and health status (UNDP 2004).

Indoor air pollution in India

India relies heavily on the use of biomass fuels for cooking and heating and there are a growing number of studies aimed at quantifying the effects of the indoor pollution produced by these sources of particulates. There is an established body of evidence on the exposure–response relationships for particulate air pollution that have been derived for outdoor air pollution in high income country urban situations, but they may not be suitable for use in low and middle income countries, particularly in rural areas.

Read the following extract by Smith (2000) on the burden of disease attributable to indoor air pollution in India.

 ### National burden of disease in India from indoor air pollution

If verified, the ill health estimated here from indoor air pollution is a substantial portion of the national total in India, 4.2–6.1%. It is equivalent to 6.3–9.2% of the burden for women and children under 5, who make up about 44% of the population but bear about two-thirds of the disease burden. . . . indoor air pollution would seem to classify as a major cause of ill health in India for it rivals or exceeds Tuberculosis, Ischemic Heart Disease, all cancers, road accidents, or all of the 'tropical' diseases combined. On a risk factor basis, the burden of dirty air at the household level lies behind only dirty water at the household level (poor water/sanitation/hygiene = 10%) and poor food at the household level (malnutrition = 22%), the largest two risk factors in India in the early 1990s. . . . it apparently substantially exceeded other major risk factors, such as hypertension, alcohol, unsafe sex, and tobacco . . . by any standard, indoor air quality would seem to be a major health issue in the country. Adding urban outdoor pollution, the total would be even greater. Taking the dubious but simple approach of adding the estimates, the total annual deaths would be 600 000–750 000. Assuming a similar mix of morbidity and mortality, the total burden from air pollution in India would be 5.9–9.2% of the total NBD, nearly rivalling poor water/sanitation/hygiene, although still well below malnutrition.

Discussion and conclusion

At the global level, India seems to have some 30% of all household solid-fuel stoves, although the estimates are generally much less reliable than in India where fuel use is determined in the national census. On that basis, the total world health impact on women and children would be roughly three times larger than the Indian estimates. A large fraction undoubtedly occurs in China, where application of broad-brush methods have also derived large health impacts of indoor and outdoor pollution with relatively more Chronic obstructive airways disease and lung cancer and less Acute Respiratory Infection than found in India . . . By themselves, epidemiological studies do not prove causality, only association. Nevertheless, when a number of studies find similar associations in different populations, places, and times; in situations of different mixes of confounders; and done by different investigators with different methods; the argument for causality starts to become stronger. The case for causality is not helped, however, by the current poor understanding of the actual physiological mechanisms that link airborne particles with ill health. The studies in less developed country solid-fuel-using households reviewed here have generally not directly measured exposures, nor have they been as nearly as extensive or sophisticated as those in developed-country urban settings. Nevertheless, particularly for the diseases above, a number of studies have been done by different investigators in different countries that found similar results. Combined with the evidence that the average particle levels in such households often reach 1 000–2 000 $\mu g/m^3$ PM_{10}, their results seem qualitatively consistent with the developed-country studies, which have been done at levels below 150 $\mu g/m^3$. On the other hand, given that most actually measured the risk of solid fuel use, there may be risks to health in addition to air pollution, perhaps through the physical burden of harvesting such fuels. The estimates made here should be viewed as tentative. They rely on distressingly few studies and many untested assumptions. Their alarming scale, however, argues for additional efforts to understand and ameliorate the conditions that lead to such severe pollution levels in the village and urban slum homes of India and elsewhere in the Third World. At the very least, they call for a serious effort to conduct the medical and abatement research that would pin down more accurately the impact of the pollution and effective ways to reduce it. Over the next decade, millions of lives may depend on it.

Activity 9.3

What difficulties did the author highlight in using epidemiological studies to understand the burden of indoor air pollution in low and middle income countries?

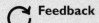 **Feedback**

The national burden of disease in India from indoor pollution has been studied by combining exposures, risks and background rates. The author points out that epidemiological studies can point to association, but not causality. However, the mounting evidence from different regions and countries strengthen the argument for the existence of a link between indoor pollution and ill health. Exposure was not directly measured, unlike studies on outdoor pollution in high income countries. Where indoor exposures have been measured, they are much greater than those in outdoor studies in high income countries. Any estimate of the burden of disease from biomass fuel should also take into consideration the added risks from the physical burden of harvesting or collecting the biomass fuel. The estimates in this study come from only a few cases with untested assumptions. The problem is large in scale and more research should be done to ascertain the impact on health.

Reducing indoor air pollution from biomass fuels

Ways to reduce the exposure of women and children to indoor particulates are listed below:

- change fuel type – processed fuels and biogas are less polluting than raw fuel, but are more expensive
- change stove type; use technology to improve energy efficiency of the stove or heater – there are relatively inexpensive alternatives available (Figure 9.3 gives an example)

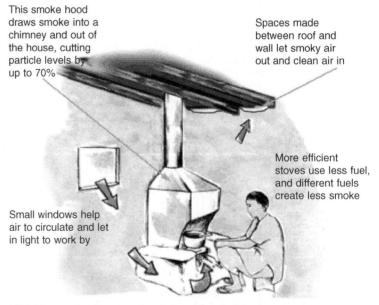

Figure 9.3 Using technology to reduce indoor air pollution
Source: http://www.itdg.org/images/smoke-diagram.gif

- separate cooking from other activities, although if space is limited this might not be possible
- reduce exposure by improving ventilation
- remove the dust in the room frequently.

Each intervention has a cost and these will need to be taken into account. You might also like to consider the roles and responsibilities of industry to provide solutions.

The indoor environment in context

Indoor activities, for example, the production of household wastes, impact upon the outdoor environment. Burning coal and biomass fuels and the disposal of sewage and waste are other important contributory factors to outdoor air pollution, particularly in low and middle income countries.

The indoor environment also has an impact upon mental health. For example, poor quality housing, over-crowding, and the threat from flooding can all influence the mental health of the inhabitants.

Summary

This chapter concentrated on the domestic indoor environment. Good quality housing can have a significant impact on improving health outcomes. You read how reducing exposure to cold housing reduced the number of excess winter deaths. Indoor air pollution is a significant environmental health concern, especially in low and middle income countries, with women and children as the most vulnerable populations due to the time they spend indoors, exposed to high levels of pollutants in confined spaces. The use of biomass fuels with inadequate ventilation is of particular concern, although substituting traditional technology with modern innovations can result in continued or even increased pollution from new sources.

References

DETR (2003) Risk rating: http://www.odpm.gov.uk/stellent/groups/odpm_housing/ documents/page/odpm_house_024525.pdf

Gupta A and Asher M (1998) *Environment and the Developing World: Principles, Policies and Management.* Chichester: John Wiley & Sons Ltd.

Howden-Chapman P (2002) Housing and inequalities in health. *Journal of Epidemiology and Community Health* 56(9): 645–6.

Howden-Chapman P, Pene G, Crane J et al. (2000) Open houses and closed rooms: Tokelau housing in New Zealand. *Health Education & Behaviour* 27(3): 351–62.

Peat JK, Dickerson J and Li J (1998) Effects of damp and mould in the home on respiratory health: a review of the literature. *Allergy* 53(2): 120–8.

Schwela D (1996) Health effects of and exposure to indoor air pollution in developing countries. In Yoshizawa S et al (eds) Indoor Air '96: proceedings of the 7th International Conference on Indoor Air Quality and Climate, Nagoya, Japan, 21–26 July, Tokyo, Institute of Public Health.

Smith, KR (2000) National burden of disease in India from indoor air pollution. *Proceedings of the National Academy of Sciences*. 21 November, 97(24).

UNDP (2004) Joint WHO/UNDP statement on indoor air pollution: www.undp.org/energy/docs/indoorairpollution.doc

UNDP/DESA/WEC (2004) *World Energy Assessment Overview: 2004 Update*. New York: UNDP.

WHO (1989) *Health Principles of Housing*. Geneva: WHO.

WHO (1995) *Concern for Europe's Tomorrow: Health and Environment*. Geneva: WHO.

Wilkinson P, Armstrong B, Landon M et al. (2001) *Cold Comfort: The Social and Environmental Determinants of Excess Winter Death in England, 1986–1996*. Bristol: The Policy Press.

World Bank (1993) *World Development Report: Investing in Health*. New York: Oxford University Press.

Further reading

Howden-Chapman P (2004) Housing standards: a glossary of housing and health. *Journal of Epidemiology and Community Health* 58(3): 162–8.

Smoke in the kitchen: health impacts of indoor air pollution in low and middle income countries: http://www.undp.org/energy/event-smk0205.htm

SECTION 3

Global issues

10 Global climate change and human health

Overview

Large-scale and global environmental hazards to human health are becoming increasingly apparent. These include climate change; stratospheric ozone depletion; loss of biodiversity; changes in hydrological systems; changes in supplies of freshwater; land degradation and stresses on food-producing systems. Appreciation of the effects of these health hazards requires an understanding of ecosystems, their complexity of these systems and how we interact with them. The effects of these changes are not distributed evenly around the world with some areas more vulnerable than others, especially among low and middle income countries that are not prepared for potential environmental impacts, and even less for health-related impacts.

Learning objectives

By the end of this chapter, you will be better able to:

- **describe the mechanisms by which global climate change may affect human health**
- **give examples of the health impact of climate change, in particular malaria, diarrhoea and problems associated with heat waves**
- **consider the physical, ethical and scientific issues raised by human-induced climate change**
- **discuss the uncertainties surrounding the impact of climate change**

Key terms

El Niño A warming of the ocean surface off the western coast of South America that occurs every four to twelve years.

Forcing agents Any phenomenon that forces the climate to change, either natural (sunlight intensity) or man-made (pollution).

Geographic Information System (GIS) An information system used to store, view, and analyse geographical information.

Greenhouse gas emissions Gases partially or wholly produced by human activity – carbon dioxide, methane, nitrogen oxides and chlorofluorocarbons (CFCs).

Remote sensing The measurement or acquisition of information from a distance, for example, the use of satellite images to study changes in waterways.

What is climate change?

The world's climate is being altered as a consequence of human activity. This has caused an increase in the atmospheric concentration of energy-trapping gases, leading to an amplification of the greenhouse effect which keeps our planet warm and habitable. The relationship between climate change and human health is very complex. There are direct impacts, such as temperature-related illness and death including the health impacts of extreme weather events; and the effect of air polluting spores and moulds. Other impacts are more indirect and lead to water- and food-borne diseases, vector-borne and rodent-borne diseases, or food and water shortages. Climate change affects ecosystem stability and biodiversity. The altering of the physical and ecological systems of the Earth is also evident through stratospheric ozone depletion, loss of biodiversity, land degradation and changes in water systems as shown in Figure 10.1. This chapter is concerned with the effects of climate change as a result of greenhouse gas emissions and the resultant warming; the other environmental issues just mentioned are discussed in more detail elsewhere in the book.

Climate change and climate variability

It is important to distinguish between the terms climate change and climate variability. Climate change is defined as a statistically significant variation in either the mean state of the climate or in its variability, persisting for an extended period (typically decades or longer) (IPCC 2001). Climate change may be due to either natural internal processes or external force. Natural processes include phenomena such as El Niño, an important factor in inter-annual climate variability. External forces include persistent human-induced changes in the composition of the atmosphere or in land use.

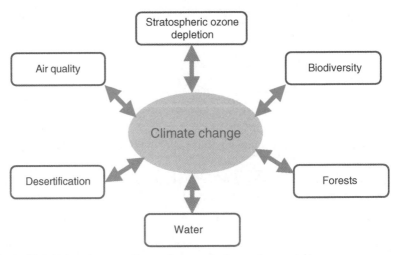

Figure 10.1 Linkage between climate change and other environmental issues
Source: Adapted from IPCC (2001)

Scientists are able to model changes in the climate using observations of past changes such as temperature, precipitation, snow and ice cover, sea level, circulation (ocean and wind currents) and extreme events. There are historical data relating to these, both directly measured and from other sources such as ice cores or tree rings. These observations can then be used in combination with mathematical modelling to simulate what may occur in the future to natural vegetation, affecting forcing agents, global climate, regional climate and occasioning high impact events.

The latest (and third) report by the Intergovernmental Panel on Climate Change (IPCC) summarizes the current scientific knowledge on how the climate may change, given future greenhouse gas emissions. The report estimates changes in the global mean temperature of between 1.4° and 5.8°C by the year 2100. International policy makers aim at maintaining the increase in warming below a 2°C threshold (global mean temperature); you will read more about the politics of climate change later in the chapter. The main findings from the IPCC suggest that the warming effect will cause a rise in sea levels and an increase in extreme weather events; the findings are summarized below:

- surface temperature is projected to rise by 1.4° to 5.8°C as a global average from 1990–2100
- the warming (thermal expansion) of the oceans, together with the melting of glaciers and ice on land, will cause a rise in sea levels round the world – mean sea level has a projected increase of 0.09 to 0.88 metres between 1990 and 2100; this will continue even after the atmospheric greenhouse gas concentrations are stabilized
- extreme weather events such as heat waves, droughts and floods are predicted to increase, as well as higher minimum temperatures and fewer cold days
- glaciers and ice caps are projected to continue their widespread retreat during the twenty-first century, with tropical and subtropical glaciers retreating the most and in some cases disappearing (IPCC 2001).

The origin of greenhouse gases

The atmosphere of the Earth admits electromagnetic radiation (including visible light from the sun) to the surface; some of this (short-wave) light energy is absorbed and then re-emitted as (long-wave) heat (see Figure 10.2). The heat retained causes a natural greenhouse effect. If there was no heat trapped by the atmosphere, the Earth's surface would be too cold to support life and all of our water would freeze. The atmosphere has been slowly changing during the past four million years.

There have been natural cycles of warming and cooling associated with fluctuating levels of carbon dioxide and methane in the atmosphere over at least the past 160,000 years. At the time of the Industrial Revolution 200 years ago, more greenhouse gases began to be emitted into the atmosphere as a result of human activity; this rise became more marked in the 1950s and has risen steadily since then (Figure 10.3). The greenhouse gases, some of which are produced by human activity, are carbon dioxide, methane, nitrogen oxides and chlorofluorocarbons

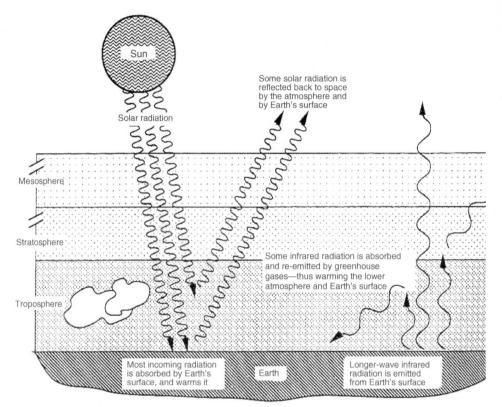

Figure 10.2 Simple version of the greenhouse effect

Source: McMichael (1993)

(CFCs), the later being entirely man-made. Although the rise in temperature during the past 100 years cannot be unquestionably attributed to human activity, the enormous increases in potentially warming greenhouse gases certainly can be, and even small rises in temperature can cause ecological havoc.

Global distribution of climate change

The effects of climate change will not be the same everywhere, for instance, not all populations would reasonably expect to run the risk of coastal flooding. Flooding caused by storm surges already affects 50 million people a year. If the sea rises by half a metre, this number could double. The low-lying oceanic nations are particularly vulnerable. For example, if the sea rises by a metre, then 1 per cent of Egypt's land, 6 per cent of the Netherlands and 17.5 per cent of Bangladesh would be inundated, and only 20 per cent of the Marshall Islands would be left above water. Other effects on human health will also be unequally distributed, as you will read in the next section. The effects of global warming are not just due to the unequal

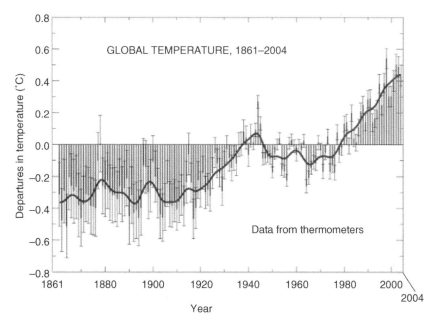

Figure 10.3 Past changes in global mean temperatures

Source: http://www.metoffice.com/research/hadleycentre/CR_data/Annual/HadCRUG.gif

distribution of the consequences, but also due to the ability of the affected countries to cope with environmental and health changes.

Direct and indirect effects on human health

Although the effects of climate change and consequent global warming are not precisely understood, some direct effects of exposure to increased temperatures can be measured, such as increased heat-related illnesses and higher death rates associated with heat waves such as the heat wave in France in 2003. Unstable weather conditions may also lead to a higher incidence of natural disasters, such as hurricanes, cyclones, drought and forest fires, which impact on the physical *and* mental health of affected communities. The pathways by which climate change may affect human health are outlined in Figure 10.4.

The altered weather patterns also have some indirect effects on human health. The effect on rainfall patterns, with increased incidence of flooding, may lead to a rise in both intestinal diseases because of its effect on water and waste provisions, and in malarial illness and other diseases caused by water-borne vectors. These indirect effects are most serious in the poorer areas of the world. The effects of climate change on heat waves and communicable diseases, particularly malaria and diarrhoea, will be considered in more detail.

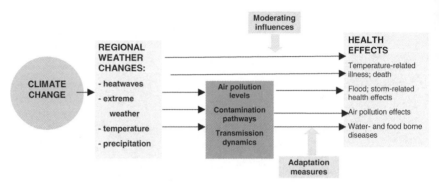

Figure 10.4 Pathways by which climate may affect human health
Source: Based on Patz and Kovats (2002)

Communicable disease and climate change

There are a number of diseases whose prevalence is predicted to increase as a result of climate change. The WHO has looked at the common diseases and identified those most likely to be affected by climate change and result in epidemic outbreaks (WHO 2004). It has been recommended that an early warning system be put in place to monitor changes in disease distribution. Table 10.1 lists some examples of the diseases with the strongest evidence for a link with climate factors.

Some non-epidemic diseases also have an association with climate change. The use of Geographical Information System (GIS) technology and remote sensing is increasingly allowing the creation of risk maps for some diseases such as intestinal nematodes. There is little seasonal variation in infection rates for these helminths, but there is some evidence that soil humidity is important (WHO 2004) and this may be affected by changing temperatures and precipitation. Geographical risk mapping of schistosomiasis, filariasis and Chagas disease have all been undertaken using data on temperature, precipitation and vegetation. Lyme disease is spread by the *ixodid* tick vector and the environmental factors that affect the distribution of ticks are well understood; this has allowed detailed mapping of the distribution. There is a peak in the summer months (Orloski, in WHO 2004), but no evidence that this is climate-related, rather that it is due to the increased likelihood of humans being outdoors in the warmer months.

Diarrhoeal disease

Diarrhoeal disease is a significant global cause of illness and death; two million children die each year in low and middle income countries despite the increasing use of oral rehydration therapy. Of all deaths associated with unsafe water, sanitation and hygiene, 99.8 per cent occur in low and middle income countries and 90 per cent of those who die are children. It does, however, remain a problem for

Table 10.1 Selected common communicable diseases, their distribution, epidemic potential and sensitivity to climate

Disease	Global Burden (1000 DALYs)	Transmission	Distribution	Evidence for interannual variability[1]	Climate – epidemic link	Strength of climate sensitivity[2]
Diarrhoeal disease	62 227 (incl. cholera)	Food- and water-borne transmission	World-wide	***	Increases in temperature and decreases in rainfall associated with epidemics. Sanitation and human behaviour are probably more important.	**
Cholera	(see diarrhoeal diseases)	Food- and water-borne transmission	Africa, Asia, South America, Russia	*****	Increases in sea and air temperatures as well as El Niño events associated with epidemics. Sanitation and human behaviour also are important.	*****
Malaria	40 213	Transmitted by the bite of female Anopheles mosquitoes	Currently endemic in >100 countries throughout the tropics and subtropics	*****	Changes in temperature and rainfall associated with epidemics. Many other locally relevant factors include vector characteristics, immunity, population movements, drug resistance, etc.	*****
Meningococcal meningitis	5 751	Air-borne transmission	World-wide	****	Increases in temperature and decreases in humidity associated with epidemics.	***
Dengue/dengue haemorrhagic fever	433	Transmitted by the bite of female Aedes mosquitoes	Africa, Europe, South America, South-East Asia, West Pacific	****	High temperature, humidity and heavy rain associated with epidemic. Non-climatic factors may have more important impact.	***
Rift Valley fever	N/A	Transmitted by the bite of female Culex and Aedes mosquitoes	Sub-Saharan Africa	***	Heavy rains associated with onset of epidemic. Cold weather associated with end of epidemic. Reservoir animal factors also are important.	***
Ross River virus	N/A	Transmitted by the bite of female Aedes and Culex mosquitoes	Australia and Pacific islands	**	High temperature and heavy precipitation associated with onset of epidemic. Host immune factors and reservoir animals also are important factors.	***

Notes: 1 – no interannual variability, * very weak variability, ** some variability, *** moderate variability, **** strong variability, ***** very strong variability
2 – no climate link, * climate link is very weak, ** climate plays a moderate role, *** climate plays a significant role, **** climate is an important factor, ***** climate is the primary factor in determining at least some epidemics, and the strength of the association between climate and disease outbreaks has been assessed on the basis of published quantitative (statistical) rather than anecdotal evidence.
Source: Adapted from WHO (2004)

high income as well as low and middle income countries, as diarrhoeal disease is not just associated with unsafe water and sanitation, but also with hygiene and food safety practices.

There has been a seasonal variation observed in the occurrence of diarrhoeal disease, with rising temperature associated with hospital admissions for diarrhoeal disease in all parts of the world. A Peruvian study found that hospital admissions increased by 4 per cent for each degree C rise in temperature in hot months, rising to 12 per cent per °C in the cool months. In Fiji a similar study found that monthly cases increased by 3 per cent per °C (Singh et al. 2001).

Climate change is predicted to impact on diarrhoeal diseases such as cholera, because changes in rainfall cause floods and monsoons which lead to seasonal epidemics and drought. These changes will also affect the supply of safe drinking water and adequate sanitation as well as the provision of safe food and the ability to put good hygiene practices in place.

High income countries report an increase of reported food poisoning in the hotter summer months. Salmonella is the second most common cause of food poisoning in England and Wales with 30–40 000 notifications per year; as this is only the number confirmed by laboratory testing, there are many more cases that go unrecorded. The salmonella bacterium grows on food at ambient temperatures and exhibits a linear relationship with temperature above a threshold of around 7–8 °C. Proper food storage involving adequate refrigeration slows or stops the growth. The disease is also spread through person-to-person contact as the result of poor hygiene behaviour. Outbreaks of salmonella are often related to poor food handling practices and hygiene, as well as to failings in the food industry. The evidence is weak that climate change will increase salmonella or other diarrhoeal diseases such as campylobacter, except through the mechanism of increased temperatures allowing greater opportunity for bacteria growth. The higher summer temperatures may lead to more opportunity for risky behaviour such as picnics, as the spread of the disease is related to food handling practices.

Malaria

Malaria is a disease caused by a parasite that is transmitted from person to person by the female *Anopheles* mosquito; it causes acute bouts of fever which may recur (see Chapter 7 for more detail on transmission and the disease burden of malaria). There are 1.1 million deaths each year as a result of malaria, mostly in children. Malaria is also responsible for 40 million Disability Adjusted Life Years (DALYs) each year. There has already been a resurgence of malaria in some areas due to drug and insecticide resistance.

You have read about the likely environmental consequences of climate change and the problems associated with malaria. Climate change may affect the spread of malaria by:

- increasing its *distribution*. Where epidemic malaria is currently limited by temperature, it may become present in new areas
- decreasing the *distribution* where it becomes too dry for mosquitoes to be sufficiently abundant for transmission

- increasing or decreasing the months of transmission
- increasing the risk of local outbreaks in areas where disease is eradicated but vectors are still present, for example, in the UK or the USA.

Modelling the distribution of malaria

Modelling is being increasingly used to help predict the effects of climate change on human health and has proved very useful in estimating the spread of malaria. The distribution of the malaria vector can be modelled and its transmission potential can be estimated as a function of climate change. There are some population and geographical groups who are more vulnerable than others to the effects of malaria. Identifying the population at particular risk is essential for public health planning. Their relative risk is expressed in terms of additional or excess cases or deaths per year, and DALYs and the costs involved can be modelled. Figure 10.5 gives an example of a theoretical model of malaria distribution in Africa. Different climate change scenarios can then be included in order to predict changes in distribution.

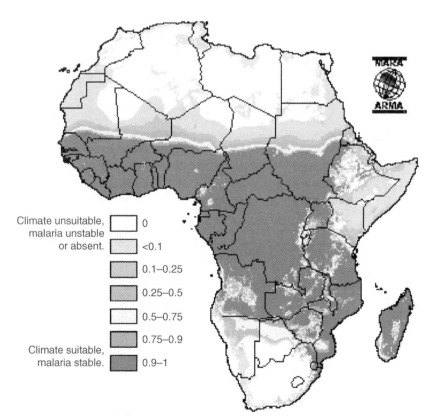

Figure 10.5 Theoretical model of malaria distribution in Africa

Source: www.mara.org.za/images/picdistr.gif

Physical changes in the environment

Climate change projections from the IPCC (2001) have estimated an increase in surface temperature ranging from 1.6° to 6°C from 1990 to 2100 and a rise in sea level ranging from 14 to 80 cm. This could prove to be a significant problem in low-lying parts of the world, as more than half of the world's population lives within 60 km of the sea. Some of the most vulnerable regions are the Nile delta in Egypt and the Ganges–Brahmaputra delta in Bangladesh; this area alone has a population of 135 million threatened by sea-level rise. There are also many small islands under threat including the Marshall Islands and the Maldives.

The Pacific Ocean contains many low-lying islands. Temperature increases and a rise in sea level are occurring in this area at a rate faster than the global average. The most immediate threat to these small island nations comes from the extreme climate variability due to El Niño. This affects rainfall patterns and moisture distribution and contributes to drought and storm events. Sea levels rise due to thermal expansion of the oceans and glacial melting will lead to the direct inundation of low-lying areas, shore erosion, exacerbation of coastal flooding and storm damage, contamination of estuaries and aquifers, destruction of coral reefs and fisheries and will threaten water resources and agriculture due to salination of freshwater aquifers (WHO 2000). The extract outlines how small island nations can prepare for the effects of sea-level rise.

 Strategies for adaptation to sea-level rise

Strategies for adaptation to sea-level rise fall into three main categories: retreat, accommodate, and protect. Retreat indicates the planned abandonment of land to reduce risk and minimize loss of associated infrastructure. In the Pacific Islands, this could mean abandoning some low-level islands or abandoning low-level areas and moving to higher ground, if available on the same island. Accommodation suggests changing land use as water levels rise such as raising buildings or changing to more salt-tolerant crops. Protection often uses constructed barriers to keep the sea away from coastlines.

'Hard' structures such as seawalls and breakwaters have traditionally been used for protection. These 'hard' structures, however, can cause additional erosion to adjacent unprotected coastal areas. Other approaches, which may be more practical and efficient for small island states, include 'softer' options such as the use of vegetation to stabilize beaches. Adding sand and stone to existing beaches, termed 'nourishment', or raising the height of some coastal villages may be useful in some places. Precautionary approaches such as the enforcement of enlarged building setbacks, land-use regulations, and building codes are gaining popularity.

The chapter on disasters (Chapter 12) includes more detail on extreme weather events related to climate change such as floods and storms and discusses the preparation of disaster plans for this type of event in more detail.

Heatwaves

Climate change has been predicted to increase the incidence and severity of extreme weather events. Over the past few years, the northern hemisphere has experienced a number of extreme heatwaves in the summer months. These were

Table 10.2 Deaths attributed to the heatwave in August 2003 in Europe

Country	Heat-stroke deaths	Excess deaths (%)	Time period	Method for estimating baseline mortality
England/Wales	§	2 045 (16)	4 to 13 August	Deaths for same period in years 1998 to 2002
France	§	14 802 (60)	1 to 20 August	Average of deaths for same period in years 2000–02
Italy	§	3 134 (15)	1 June to 15 August	Deaths in same period in 2002
Portugal	7	2 099 (26)	1 to 31 August	Deaths in same period in 97–01
Spain	59	?		–
The Netherlands	§	400–650	1 to 3 August	

Note: § not reported
Source: Kovats et al. (2004)

responsible for thousands of excess deaths and tested the ability of the authorities and the infrastructure to cope. Many of the excess deaths in heatwaves or cold waves occur in people with pre-existing disease. The true impact of heatwaves is difficult to determine as the deaths of many of the susceptible individuals, the elderly, frail, or very young have been brought forward by a few days or week. See the extract on harvesting in Chapter 9 for a more detailed explanation of this phenomenon. If changes in the global climate lead to an increase in these events of temperature extremes, then governments and other agencies will need to ensure that essential services and infrastructure can adapt to cope. The freak heatwave in 2003 provides an example of the consequences of poor planning for extreme weather events. France seemed to be particularly badly affected in the August heatwave compared to other countries with a 14,802 extra deaths (60 per cent) compared to the same period in the years 2000–02 (see Table 10.2).

System failures which may have contributed to the death toll included a sur-veillance system which did not register the actual number of deaths occurring in a timely way because it was not designed to register this form of change in death rates; institutional failures including lack of emergency planning in the health service; poor meteorological forecasts which did not predict the heatwave, or the length of time it was likely to continue. Overall there was no real experience or knowledge of this type of event in this area and no public health measures had been put into place to try and mitigate the effects.

🖊 Activity 10.1

You have been asked by the health department of your government to begin to make a public health plan for extreme weather events. Your task is to note the information you need to find and the processes or stages you will have to go through in order to assess the impact on health of extreme weather events.

Feedback

Your health plan might have included any of the following considerations (Kovats et al. 2003):

- evaluate the impact of climate variability and change (taking account of vulnerable populations, and total burdens)
- evaluate possible threshold effects
- evaluate the effects of multiple stresses, including changes in socioeconomic systems
- evaluate uncertainty and its implications for risk management
- evaluate the effects of reducing emissions (impacts of stabilization scenarios)
- measure coping capacity, especially under different socioeconomic futures

The assessment process should do the following:

- balance near-term and long-term effects
- weigh the different potential effects in different population groups
- balance the more certain, quantifiable potential effects with those that are less certain and not quantifiable, as well as the qualitative effects
- balance the interests of the various stakeholder groups: experts, people potentially affected and decision makers

Uncertainties of climate change scenarios

The effects of climate change have been modelled using a range of different scenarios (Table 10.3). Each of these are plausible and self-consistent descriptions of the future global climate but have used different assumptions and have uncertainties in their estimates.

Table 10.3 Main effects on health of global climate change

	Effect
Direct	Deaths, illness and injury due to exposure to heatwaves Effects on the respiratory system Climate-related disasters, cyclones, floods, droughts, fires
Indirect	Altered spread and transmission of vector-borne diseases such as malaria Altered transmission of contagious diseases, for example, cholera and influenza Disturbance and impairment of crop production due to effects on soil, water, temperature and pests Various consequences of sea-level rise which include inundations, sewerage disruption, soil salinity and loss of biodiversity Demographic disruption, environmental refugees

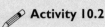 **Activity 10.2**

What are some of the uncertainties associated with modelling of climate change?

Feedback

The main sources of uncertainty are:

- unknown future greenhouse gas emissions
- natural climate variability
- different responses between different global climate models
- poorly resolved regional and local climate changes
- possibility of abrupt, non-linear changes in the climate system

The existence of uncertainties does not imply the absence of knowledge; we under-stand some aspects of future climate change better than others. For example, there is more confidence in the models of future increases in carbon dioxide concentrations and mean sea level than in modelled increases in storms or a higher incidence of summer droughts. The likelihood of a rapid and non-linear change in regional climates is not able to be quantified using current data.

The politics of climate change

Because greenhouse gas emissions affect the entire globe, it means that the international community has had to meet to try to resolve the issues involved in limiting their effect. So far, the main contributors to global warming have been the rich industrialized nations, although the poorer nations are rapidly following in their footsteps with increased industrial pollution and an enormous increase in the use of private transport. As we have seen, economic development is associated with an increase in energy use. The Earth Summit in 1992 emphasized the need for international cooperation on climate change. This was followed up with a number of meetings including the 1997 meeting in Kyoto at which the Kyoto Protocols were drafted. Article 2 of the United Nations Framework Convention on Climate Change agrees that change is needed. It states that:

> The ultimate objective of this Convention and any related legal instruments that the Conference of the Parties may adopt is to achieve, in accordance with the relevant provisions of the Convention, stabilization of greenhouse gas concentrations in the atmosphere at a level that would prevent dangerous anthropogenic interference with the climate system. Such a level should be achieved within a time frame sufficient to allow ecosystems to adapt naturally to climate change, to ensure that food production is not threatened and to enable economic development to proceed in a sustainable manner.

The Kyoto Protocol was signed by 150 nations, but left some of the details to be worked out later, and this is still ongoing. In 2001, President George W. Bush decided not to sign the protocol. This was a significant setback as the USA is the major source of greenhouse gas emissions. The protocol was finally ratified in October 2004 when Russia signed, and it came into force in February 2005. The main thrust of the Kyoto Protocol was to reduce net emissions to 5 per cent below the 1990 levels. In the first commitment period between 2008 and 2012, some countries have lower targets, and Australia, if it signed the protocol, would be allowed increased emissions.

The IPCC Third Assessment Report has now established that low and middle income countries are most at risk from climate change, although the emissions are still relatively low. Setting targets to reduce climate change is about providing equity for low and middle income nations, and ensuring sustainable development now and in the future.

The targets set in the Kyoto Protocol can be achieved in a number of ways. Countries can reduce emissions by changing the technologies used, by making use of energy-efficient processes and by changing the energy economy from carbon-based fuels to hydrogen, wind and other renewable sources. This can be achieved by carbon trading whereby allowances of carbon emissions are bought and sold, often between developed and developing countries. Any carbon traded can come from that which is already permitted for emission, from any reductions in emissions (via new technology, energy efficiency, renewable energy), or can be offset against emissions, for example, via carbon sequestration (capture of carbon in biomass such as forests). The first carbon trade took place in March 2003 between Shell, the global oil company, and Nuon (a Dutch-based multinational that supplies power to users in Belgium and Germany), in which Nuon bought a significant volume of allowances from Shell for 2005.

Article 12 of the protocol also supports the Clean Development Mechanism, which allows high income countries to assist low and middle income countries in using cleaner energy sources such as solar panels. If Clean Development Mechanism projects result in 'certified emission reductions', then the high income country can use the certified emission reduction to comply with their own quantified emissions reduction commitments.

Climate change and sustainable development

The potential consequences of climate change are a significant challenge to the environment, the global economy, and human health, with changes affecting future generations. Sustainable development is crucial to the success of climate change mitigation. However, it is not just future generations that are at risk; some communities are already experiencing the effects of climate change such as small islands, developing states and the high Arctic in particular. Action on climate change requires:

- a focus on equity and sustainable development by working at different levels
- constructive engagement at the international level
- strong national policies as well as action by individuals.

Equity

Climate change will not have an equal effect across the environment and the different populations of the globe. The USA currently produces 25 per cent of the annual greenhouse gas emissions, yet has only 5 per cent of the world population. The ability of a country or a region to cope with climate change depends on its wealth, technology and infrastructure. Low and middle income countries do not have the industry, transportation, or intensive agricultural practices that are the cause of global warming. However, they have limited capacity to protect themselves against the adverse consequences and as you have read, may be particularly vulnerable to the effects, for example, sea-level rises would affect Bangladesh and low-lying Pacific islands.

Dealing with climate change is a challenge for environmental and health equity. Choosing not to use what is often more expensive, energy-efficient technology will decrease the imbalance of 'equity' at least in the short term, but will increase the problems of global warming (Patz and Kovats 2002).

The IPCC recognizes that sustainable development is a key factor in climate change mitigation (Figure 10.6). In order to succeed in the long term, policies and actions will need to work with other environmental protection initiatives, promote economic growth and enhance social equity.

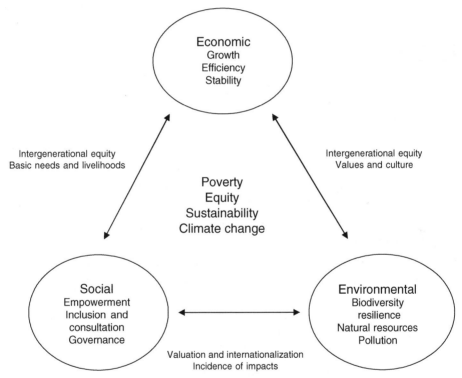

Figure 10.6 Key elements of sustainable development and interconnections
Adapted from IPCC (2001)
Source: http://www.ipcc.ch/present/graphics/2001syr/small/00.22.jpg

---

✏ **Activity 10.3**

What are the main moral, political and scientific problems associated with human-induced climate change?

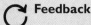 **Feedback**

As you will have noted, the first moral issue is the bequest to future generations of an ecologically damaged world. The second is that although the change has been caused mainly by the rich industrial countries, the entire world will suffer – and the poorer countries are likely to suffer the most.

The main political issue arises from the last point: the poorer countries are entitled to industrialize but cannot afford the expensive technology needed to do so in an environmentally protective manner. If the whole world is to benefit from economic development, the rich countries will have to aid the poorer countries in order to prevent an even greater build-up of greenhouse gases.

The scientific problem arises from the uncertainty inherent in the data: it is not known precisely how great a cutback in energy use is required to bring about a stabilization or reversal of the climatic damage believed to have been caused so far.

Summary

In this chapter, you explored one of the main global health issues, that of climate change. The probable cause of climate change appears to be human-induced and there are a number of direct and indirect health consequences. The Kyoto Protocol aims to reduce the amount of carbon emissions and slow the effect of global warming. You also read of the importance of sustainable development and equity in achieving results and the uncertainties in making estimates of the effects.

References

IPCC Intergovernmental Panel on Climate Change (2000) *Special Report on Methodological and Technological Issues in Technology Transfer*. Metz B, Davidson OR, Martens JM, van Rooijen S and van Wie McGrory L (eds). New York: Cambridge University Press.

IPCC (2001) *Climate Change 2001: Impacts, Adaptation and Vulnerability*. Report of Working Group II to the Intergovernmental Panel on Climate Change Third Assessment Report. McCarthy JJ, Canziani OF, Leary NA, Dokken DJ and White KS (eds). New York: Cambridge University Press.

Kovats RS, Ebi K and Menne B (2003) *Methods of Assessing Human Health Vulnerability and Public Health Adaptation to Climate Change*. WHO, Health Canada, UNEP, WMO, Copenhagen. (Health and Global Environmental Change Series, No. 1). http://www.euro.who.int/document/E81923.pdf

Kovats S, Wolf T and Menne B (2004) Heatwave of August 2003: provisional estimates of the impact on mortality. *Eurosurveillance Weekly* 8(11): http://www.eurosurveillance.org/ew/2004/040311.asp#7

McMichael AJ (1993) *Planetary Overload: Global Environmental Change and the Health of the Human Species*. Cambridge: Cambridge University Press.

Patz JA and Kovats RS (2002) Hot spots in climate change and human health. *British Medical Journal* 325: 1094–8.

Singh RBK, Hales S, de Wet N et al. (2001) The influence of climate variation and change on diarrhoeal disease in the Pacific Islands. *Environmental Health Perspectives* 109(2): 155–9.

WHO (2000) Workshop report: climate variability and change and their health effects in Pacific Island countries. Apia, Samoa, 25–28 July.

WHO (2004) *Using Climate to Predict Disease Outbreaks: A Review*: WHO/SDE/OEH/04.01 2004.

Further reading

Eco equity, campaigning for equal rights to global common resources: http://www.ecoequity.org/

IISD Linkages, resource for environment and development policy makers: http://www.iisd.ca/

Intergovernmental Panel on Climate Change: http://www.ipcc.ch/

McMichael AJ, Campbell-Lendrum D, Corvalan C, Ebi KL, Githeko AK, Scheraga JS, and Woodward A (eds) (2003) *Climate Change and Health: Risks and Responses*. Geneva: WHO. www.who.int/globalchange/climate

Tóth F. (ed) (1999) *Fair Weather: Equity Concerns in Climate Change*. London: EarthScan.

Tyndall Centre for Climate Change Research: http://www.tyndall.ac.uk/

United Nations Framework Convention on Climate Change: http://unfccc.int/

11   The balance of ecosystems and human health

Overview

A change in the environmental conditions in one part of the world can lead to a reaction in another part of the world (this is called the butterfly effect). Our environmental problems do not necessarily stop at regional or national boundaries, but frequently have consequences elsewhere. One of the results of this is global climate change and there are other consequences which include stratospheric ozone depletion, acidic precipitation and loss of biodiversity.

Learning objectives

By the end of this chapter, you will be better able to:

- **discuss the direct and indirect consequences of stratospheric ozone depletion on human health**
- **explain the range of consequences of acidic precipitation**
- **assess how the ecological system is affected by loss of biodiversity**
- **give examples of how changes in the ecosystem can affect human health**

Key terms

Acidic precipitation Acidic chemicals dissolved in rainwater and other precipitations.

Stratospheric ozone depletion Reduction of ozone in the stratosphere.

Ultraviolet (UV) radiation Invisible electromagnetic radiation from sunlight.

Ozone depletion and ultraviolet radiation

High in the stratosphere there is a layer of ozone molecules (trioxygen O_3), formed by the action of ultraviolet (UV) radiation on oxygen molecules (dioxygen O_2). Ozone has accumulated over a great deal of time; it acts as a screen which absorbs some of the UV radiation and prevents it from reaching the Earth's surface. Damage caused to the ozone layer by chlorofluorocarbons (CFCs) and other chemicals during the past century has thinned it, allowing more UV radiation to pass through. There is a hole in the ozone layer above Antarctica from September to December each year, and a small hole in the Arctic region, as well as some losses at middle latitudes.

The Montreal Protocol

In 1974 Molina and Rowland proposed that when CFCs were exposed to ultraviolet radiation at low temperatures they would release free chlorine radicals (Cl•) which catalyse the breakdown of ozone. CFCs were synthetic chemicals used as refrigerants, anaesthetics, solvents, propellants and in polystyrene manufacture. They had previously been seen as safe and inert chemicals.

When the research was released, it generated some controversy but it was not until 1978 that the United States became the first country to ban the use of CFCs in spray cans, followed by the European Union in 1985. The Vienna Convention declared good intent on the banning of CFCs and was signed by 20 nations. This was the first international agreement on an environmental issue to be signed before scientific data were available on the effects (McMichael 1993). This use of the pre-cautionary principle was based on theoretical prediction and the knowledge that ultraviolet radiation is biologically damaging. In 1987, 36 nations met in Montreal and agreed to restrict the release of ozone-depleting chemicals and to halve CFC emissions by 2000.

Over time, the Montreal Protocol has been amended as more scientific evidence has been confirmed. The latest version is the Beijing Amendment which came into force in 2002 (UNEP 2004). By the time of the Beijing meeting, funds were forthcoming to help the People's Republic of China and India to phase out CFCs. However, CFCs are still being produced by countries with economies in transition, and this will continue until funding can be provided to phase these out and introduce the use of suitable alternatives.

The direct effects of ozone depletion on health

The health effects of ozone depletion are both direct and indirect. Direct effects include skin cancer, eye damage and damage to the immune system. Indirect effects include damage to terrestrial and aquatic systems, which themselves generate further consequences for the environment and human health.

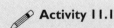 **Activity 11.1**

Read the following extract by Longstreth and colleagues (1998) and then summarize the main health effects associated with ozone depletion.

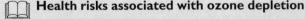 **Health risks associated with ozone depletion**

The health risks associated with ozone depletion will principally be those due to increased ultraviolet B radiation (UV-B) in the environment, i.e., increased damage to the eyes, the immune system and the skin. Some new risks may also be introduced with the increased use of alternatives to the ozone-depleting substances. Quantitative risk estimates are available for some of the UV-B-associated effects, e.g., cataracts and skin cancer; however, the data are insufficient to develop similar estimates for effects such as immuno-suppression and the toxicity of alternatives.

Ocular damage from UV exposures includes effects on the cornea, lens, iris and associated epithelial and conjunctival tissues. The most common acute ocular effect of environmental ultraviolet radiation (UVR) is photokeratitis. Also known as snowblindness in skiers, this condition also occurs in other outdoor recreationists. Chronic eye conditions likely to increase with ozone depletion include cataract, squamous cell carcinoma, ocular melanoma and a variety of corneal/conjunctival effects, e.g., pterygium and pinguecula.

Suppression of local (at the site of UV exposure) and systemic (at a distant, unexposed site) immune responses to a variety of antigens has been demonstrated in both humans and animals exposed to UV-B. In experiments with animals these effects have been shown to worsen the course/outcome of some infectious diseases and cancers. There is reasonably good evidence that such immunosuppression plays a role in human carcinogenesis; however, the implications of such immunosuppression for human infectious diseases are still unknown.

In light-skinned populations, exposure to solar UVR appears to be the most important environmental risk factor for basal and squamous cell carcinomas and cutaneous melanoma. Originally it was believed that total accumulated exposure to UVR was the most important environmental factor in determining risk for these tumors. Recent information now suggests that only squamous cell carcinoma risk is related to total exposure. In the cases of both basal cell carcinoma and melanoma, new information suggests that increases in risk are tied to early exposures (before about age 15), particularly those leading to severe sunburns.

Recent quantitative risk estimates have been developed for cataract, melanoma and all skin cancers combined. These estimates indicate that, under the Montreal adjustments, cataract, and skin cancer incidence will peak mid-century at an additional incidence of just under 3 per 100,000 and about 7 per 100,000, respectively.

 Feedback

Sunlight is important for physical health, however, too much can cause various adverse health effects such as skin cancer, premature ageing of the skin, eye disorders and suppression of the immune system. The latter two effects are important as they do not depend on skin pigmentation and can have world-wide implications. Those who are already immuno-compromised in some way through illness or malnutrition will be most affected. It is increasingly clear that excessive UV exposure should be avoided to minimize the risk of development of such disorders.

The indirect effects of ozone depletion

There is still speculation about the effects of UV-B exposure on plants and animals. There are some crops which are vulnerable to UV-B and will show a drop in yield, just as many others can adapt to UV-B radiation and could be used to develop UV-B-tolerant crops and forestry trees. The natural ecosystem has a mixture of resistant plants and some of these areas may be under threat.

Excess UV-B exposure impairs photosynthesis and growth hormones; detrimental effects accumulate over time, leading to a reduction in crop and forestry yields. Because UV-B exposure is selective in its effects, this might result in an altered plant profile, thus upsetting the Earth's ecological system. Phytoplankton, described as the 'grass of the sea', and zooplankton are also adversely affected by increased UV-B exposure as they are close to the surface. A possible decline in the zoo-plankton population would ultimately lead to a decline in general fish stocks. Animals can be affected by UV-B radiation in the same way as humans, with skin cancers forming on the non-pigmented areas of their skin.

Acidic precipitation

The effects of acidic chemicals dissolved in the rainwater, snow and other forms of precipitation can damage delicate aquatic systems as well as some species of plants and trees. These acidic chemicals, mainly oxides of sulphur and nitrogen, originate from industrial sources. This effect was first observed in 1850 around Manchester in England. This was a heavily industrialized area with significant use of coal, a rich source of sulphur dioxide emissions. These emissions may be carried very long distances in the clouds and ultimately fall as acid precipitation, hundreds or thousands of kilometres from their original source.

The effect is seen in many parts of the world, Canada has extensive problems resulting from emissions in the Midwestern USA and in Scandinavia the damage to forests is the result of emissions mainly from Germany and the UK. The main effect is upon aquatic systems and on some plants and forests. Small bodies of water in particular are unable to compensate for the changes in acidity and there is a follow-on effect on the biota such as plants, bacteria, fish and amphibians, leading to a simplification of the ecosystem. There is also mobilization of toxic chemicals such as the ions of aluminium, copper, lead and mercury into the water. Trees suffer from lack of nutrients and die off, following defoliation; this is thought to be chiefly the effect of a culmination of aluminium ions.

Direct effects on humans are more difficult to assess; there may be increased airway reactivity and asthma although this is likely to be a small effect, if any. The presence of negative health effects from the toxic metals in groundwater is suggested, but as yet unproven. There may also be a bio-accumulation of toxic metals such as mercury in fish which can then enter the human food chain.

Acid rain can also cause damage to food crops. This occurs in three ways: (1) direct damage to the crop; (2) acidification of the soil leading to diminished fertility; and (3) the leaching of heavy metals such as cadmium into the crop. The possible beneficial effect of acid rain in some areas must be acknowledged; this occurs in regions with sulphur-deficient soil; the depositing of sulphate ions in the soil may lead to a fertilizing effect (McMichael 1993).

Other environmental consequences of acidification

The pollutants that are responsible for acidification also play a role in other changes to the environment, including climate change and eutrophication. They are also a precursor for the production of ground-level ozone. Nitrogen oxides, together with volatile organic compounds, form ground-level ozone in the presence of sunlight. Ozone causes damage to agricultural crops, trees and humans, including eye irritation and respiratory tract irritation, exacerbation of respiratory disease and reduced exercise capacity. The concentration of ground-level ozone regularly reaches harmful levels all over Europe. The presence of ozone at ground level should not be confused with the effects noted earlier in this chapter about ozone in the stratosphere.

Biodiversity

Biodiversity refers to the multiplicity of species, plants and animals in a biological community and the ecological niches that they occupy. It is a fundamental principle of ecology that diversity in animal and plant species leads to greater stability of the ecosystem. This is, in part, because the ecosystem functions more efficiently with different species occupying more niches and extracting full benefit from the energy and nutrients available. An explanation for this seems to be that more complicated systems have greater adaptability in the face of environmental changes, because ecological niche occupants may overlap to some extent and allow substitutions if one or more are lost. Loss of biodiversity therefore means a less stable, less adaptable system that is able to restore itself (Yassi et al. 2001).

The World Summit on Sustainable Development in Johannesburg in 2002 recognized the importance of biodiversity in sustainable development and the eradication of poverty through the livelihood and cultural integrity of humans and the health of the planet. Biological products contribute 40 per cent to the global economy and loss of biodiversity is a direct threat to this.

 Activity 11.2

Ecosystems can have biodiversity in many ways. The following extract from the Australian government (2003) highlights threats to biodiversity hotspots in Australia.

 Preserving biodiversity in Australia

Australia is one of the most biologically diverse countries in the world, with a large portion of our species found nowhere else. But that biodiversity – the plants, animals, micro-organisms and their ecosystems – is threatened by the impact of human activities.

Biodiversity hotspots are areas under immediate threat from impacts such as salinity, land clearing, weeds and feral animals, and are strongholds for large numbers of Australia's unique plants and animals. The hotspots are home to 'endemic' species – in other words, native flora and fauna that are mostly restricted to one geographic locality . . . Since European settlement, more than 50 species of Australian animals and over 60 species of Australian plants are known to have become extinct. For example,

1. Einasleigh and Desert Uplands (Queensland)
   Current threats come from unsustainable grazing pressure, feral animals and in

some areas tree clearing. Changing fire regimes and exotic weeds which accompany more intensive grazing have the potential to affect bird species such as the endangered Buff-breasted Button-quail, now restricted to only a few sites.
2. North Kimberley (Western Australia)
This area consists mainly of Aboriginal land and pastoral grazing leases and is characterised by savanna woodland. With grazing has come changed fire regimes and a continuing general deterioration of the landscape. Extensive dry season fires have damaged sensitive tropical and sub-tropical forests and woodlands. Rainforest patches provide refuges for invertebrates, now under threat from fire and stock. Feral cats are common and feral pigs populations are expanding, while colonisation by cane toads is a future threat.

The importance of the loss of biodiversity and damage to ecosystems has been emphasized in this chapter and in Chapter 11 on climate change; how do you think the loss of biodiversity affects the ecosystem and why is this important?

Feedback

Ecosystems can lose biodiversity in many ways. Individual species may become extinct through hunting, chemical poisoning, habitat loss, or reduction in the species that they depend on for food. Entire ecosystems or vast areas of larger ecosystems may be changed or lost by urbanization and agricultural clearance, with particular habitats of individual species with limited ranges destroyed in the same ways. The essential area lost may relate to feeding requirements, territoriality or breeding. Sometimes, foreign species are introduced into a stable ecosystem, preying on and reducing the numbers of local species that give the ecosystem stability and sometimes, in the most extreme cases, all of these mechanisms occur at the same time. Whatever the cause, a narrowing of biodiversity is known to lead to ecological destabilization and the ultimate impact on the environment and human health could be disastrous.

Human health and biodiversity

Humans have been cultivating and collecting plants and animals for their own purposes for thousands of years. The identification of edible plants as well as plant substances that can treat disease, act as pesticides, or have industrial uses (such as cotton and latex) have been ongoing, and we still have not identified them all. Loss of biodiversity may threaten this source of nutrition and innovation.

Many pharmaceuticals originate from natural sources, including the antibiotic penicillin, which is a natural toxin that kills bacteria, released by particular fungal moulds. WHO has estimated that three-quarters of all primary health care is by traditional medicine (90 per cent in low and middle income countries) (McMichael 1993). Half of all prescription drugs originate from substances extracted from natural organisms. There are plant substances both from the tropics and temperate areas that have been identified as useful in the treatment of cancer.

Malaria and quinine

When European explorers and traders first went to tropical countries, especially Africa, they battled with death and disease caused by malaria. In the late seventeenth and eighteenth centuries, through a combination of accident, luck and observation, they discovered that the extract of the bark of the Peruvian cinchona tree both prevented and treated malaria. The active ingredient was identified in the nineteenth century as chloroquine. This chemical or similar has since proved the basis for most anti-malarial preparations. However, in many areas there are now chloroquine-resistant strains of *Plasmodium falciparum*. There is some ongoing research into drugs derived from *artemisinin* – extracted from a Chinese herb. It had been known for some time that this drug was useful for the treatment of fevers and it had been used by the Chinese for 2,000 years. If there is irony in the discovery of the cinchona tree in the tropics, it is that which has allowed humans to occupy and ultimately exploit the rainforest to a damaging degree.

Once a plant has been identified as useful to humans, there is a danger that it will become extinct. The cinchona tree was harvested almost to the point of extinction before the Dutch made a very successful plantation in Java that supplied 90 per cent of all quinine until the 1940s. Taxol is a potent anti-cancer drug found in the Pacific yew (*Taxux brevifolia*); this is being felled as part of commercial forestry and was being rapidly depleted. There is now an agreement by the US Government to declare it a threatened species. If sustainable forestry practices such as conservative logging and good management are employed, then the yew should be saved (McMichael 1993). It is not only plants but also animals that are a source of medicinal drugs, in particular, *bufo* toxins from various amphibians, and yet their habitats are under threat in many parts of the world.

Food and biodiversity

Biodiversity allows plant species to grow in unproductive or degraded land. The careful breeding of wild strains with domesticated stock has meant that agricultural practices can spread into new areas. Wheat, maize and rice provide half of the world's food, and new ways have been found to substantially increase yields. In some areas this has meant vast areas planted in single varieties; while this has meant increases in yield and ease of harvesting, it has also meant the potential loss of some cultivars as well as the opportunity for pest or disease outbreaks to devastate whole areas. This has occurred in Ireland (and other parts of Northern Europe) in the 1840s when over 2 million people starved to death when the potato crop failed partly due to infection with *Phytophthora infestans*.

To ensure food security, we need to preserve genetic diversity. There are now seed banks throughout the world, collecting as many different cultivars as possible and storing them.

Genetic modification (GM)

There has always been selective breeding of plants to obtain desired traits such as high yield, and resistance to pest or drought. The genetic modification of organisms using genes from other species is used to alter crop characteristics, e.g. their yield, pest resistance or herbicide tolerance. The technology is not without controversy. The arguments against genetic modification focus on the unknown health, environmental and economic risks. For example, consumers may have allergic reactions to novel substances, pest resistance or herbicide tolerance could spread into wild plants, and there could be toxicity to wildlife. Opponents are also wary of repercussions of increasing the control of agriculture by large bio-technology corporations. Arguments in favour of genetic modification include the solving of some food production problems due to the production of greater crop yields. Proponents argue that genetic modification of crops can therefore help to alleviate food shortages in low income countries.

Deforestation

Currently about 30 per cent of the Earth's land surface is forested; less than half of this is primary, undisturbed forest. The rate of destruction is increasing, particularly in the rainforests where two-thirds of the clearance is for agricultural purposes secondary to the needs of growing populations. The Millennium Goals aimed at ensuring sustainable development, include preference being given to land covered by forest. In the past ten years the proportion of land covered by forest has decreased slightly world-wide, but quite marked reductions have occurred in South-East Asia (Table 11.1).

Table 11.1 Proportion of land covered by forest

	Percentage of land area	
	1990	*2000*
Northern Africa	1.0	1.0
Sub-Saharan Africa	29.3	27.1
Caribbean	24.4	25.0
Latin America	50.4	48.0
Eastern Asia	15.4	17.0
Southern Asia	13.5	13.3
South-Eastern Asia	53.9	48.6
Western Asia	3.1	3.1
Oceania	68.0	65.7
Commonwealth of Independent States (Asia)	5.1	5.8
Commonwealth of Independent States (Europe)	48.9	49.2
Developed regions	25.7	25.9
World	30.3	29.6

Source: United Nations (2004)

Deforestation results in a loss of natural habitat and of biodiversity (Table 11.2). The effects of deforestation in tropical areas have some immediate local effects; there is increased soil erosion and resultant sedimentation of rivers with loss of plants and animals. The tropical forests have the richest ecosystems on Earth. Forests have a critical role in the removal and storage of carbon dioxide from the atmosphere, identified as being important for the regulation of global climate

Table 11.2 Consequences of tropical deforestation

Effects	Consequences
Local effects	soil erosion by gullies and slopewash small slope failures accelerated loss of sediment less infiltration and increased runoff loss of soil fertility
Regional effects	large slope failures via mass movement and debris flows increased flooding in rivers alteration of rivers characteristics coastal sediment problems loss of regional flora and fauna alteration of lifestyle of local inhabitants climatic changes
Global effects	loss of biodiversity contribution to global warming possible climate changes

Source: Gupta and Asher (1998)

change and discussed in Chapter 10. If there is increasing deforestation, then the ability to hold carbon dioxide is reduced.

Forests are being cleared for agriculture by people who have little other access to alternative economic strategies. In the short term, this provides jobs and some economic security, but this practice is difficult to regulate by governments and is not sustainable in the long term. There are a number of innovative programmes designed to reduce deforestation and preserve the forests for the future; not all of these are successful, as they rely on input and the cooperation of local and national agencies and logging companies. The extract from Gupta and Asher (1998) outlines the argument for protecting tropical forests.

 Economic harvesting and sustainability of tropical forests

The tropical forests should be preserved to meet local needs for a long time and for the rich biodiversity. It has been estimated that the total earnings from the combined harvest of forest products (including rattan, bamboo, oil latex, tannin, dyes, and pharmaceutical products) can be as high as $200 per hectare annually. This is higher than the earnings from logging and the yield may be only as high as $150 per hectare. Wildlife that attracts tourism also raises more money than logging. It is estimated that a lion in the Amboseli National Park, Kenya, brings in $27,000 per year in tourist money and the figure for a herd of elephants is $610,000. Forests also need to be preserved as important sinks for carbon, which if released to the atmosphere will accelerate global warming. In this sense sustainability of forest, irrespective of their location, is beneficial for the planet. Their management and preservation, however, require financial adjustments, product substitutions, and forest management on global to local scales.

Successful sustainable management of forests requires a combination of physical, economic, technical and political processes. Sustainable managed forests can bring in significant revenues and jobs for local people. For example, maintaining forests as part of mixed cultivation with food crops or as hedges in farmland has been successful in some parts of the world. India, in particular helps to preserve the primary forest from further decimation while still providing essential supplies of wood. Thorough environmental impact assessments are needed when large-scale mining projects are proposed. These involve clearance of large areas of forests. In some instances this involves the loss of the forest which may make the project unprofitable. In 1985 the Tropical Forest Action Plan (TFAP) was formulated and was designed to involve local communities and national governments in the management of forests. National and local policies have had mixed success (Gupta and Asher 1998).

Action on biodiversity

Progress toward sustainable development and continued human well-being relies on the ability to maintain ecosystems and biodiversity. The demands on the ecosystem for the provision of water and food are growing, but human activity has degraded many ecosystems. Good management can reverse some damage and prevent more from occurring. At the Earth Summit in Rio in 1992 the Convention on Biological Diversity was signed by 200 participating countries. It was designed to provide an international framework for biodiversity and the sustainable use and equitable sharing of the benefits. The countries at the subsequent Johannesburg Summit in 2002 agreed that action should be taken to reduce the rate of current loss of biodiversity by 2010. To achieve the targets agreed there needs to be monitoring, an understanding of the causal relationships between human activities and environmental change and the availability of options to prevent the loss of biodiversity (EEA 2004). The Millennium Ecosystem Assessment was established to improve the knowledge base, to understand the complicated relationship between ecosystems and human well-being and devise options for appropriate interventions (Millennium Assessment 2002). There has been an increase in the past 14 years in the geographical areas put aside and protected to ensure biodiversity. This is most apparent in Western Asia where the proportion of protected land has increased from 4 to 18 per cent.

Summary

This chapter has examined some of the probable causes of recent changes in the world's environment and the direct and indirect effects of this on the ecosystem and human health. Ozone depletion caused by the release in the atmosphere of CFCs and other industrial chemicals has led to eye diseases, immunological damage and cancers. While it is not presently possible to estimate with certainty the ultimate effects of the ecological damage caused by development, agriculture and industrialization, the ensuing loss of biodiversity has already impacted severely on the world's ecosystems.

References

Australian Government (2003) (http://www.deh.gov.au/minister/env/2003/mr03oct03a.html#maps) EEA (2004).

Farman J (2001) Halocarbons, the ozone layer and the precautionary principle, in Harremoes P, Gee D, McGarvin M et al. (eds) *Late Lessons from Early Warnings: The Precautionary Principle 1896–2000*. Luxembourg: Office for Official Publications of the European Communities.

Gupta A and Asher M (1998) *Environment and the Developing World: Principles, Policies and Management*. Chichester: John Wiley & Sons Ltd.

Longstreth J et al. (1998) Late lessons from early warnings: the precautionary principle 1896–2000 http://sedac.ciesin.org/ozone/docs/UNEP98/UNEP98p12.html

McMichael AJ 1993 *Planetary Overload*. Cambridge: Cambridge University Press.

Millennium Ecosystems Assessment: http://www.millenniumassessment.org/

UNEP 2004 Ozone Secretariat: http://www.unep.org/ozone/Treaties_and_Ratification/2Bi_amendments%20to%20montreal%20protocol.asp

United Nations (2004) *Implementation of the United Nations Millennium Declaration: Report of the Secretary-General*. New York: United Nations.

Yassi A, Kjellstrom T, de Kok T and Guidotti TL (2001) *Basic Environmental Health*. Oxford: Oxford University Press.

Further reading

New Scientist: http://www.newscientist.com/hottopics/gm/

Ozone maps: http://es-ee.tor.ec.gc.ca/cgi-bin/selectMap

Disasters

Overview

It is not only human beings who damage the Earth's environment, nor is the damage always as slow and insidious as the effects of pollution. Natural disasters are often sudden and immediately devastating in their impact, leaving immense environmental, health and economic costs that can match man-made disasters in scale. In the past 20 years, three million deaths have been caused by natural disasters alone; at the end of 2004 more than 273,000 people died in a single incident – the South-East Asian tsunami.

Learning objectives

By the end of this chapter, you will be better able to:

* **describe the types and causes of natural and man-made disasters, including emerging issues such as climate change**
* **understand the importance of planning for disaster relief and mitigation**
* **discuss the public health consequences of war, including refugees**

Key terms

Climatological factors Climates and their phenomena including temperature, windspeed, cloud cover, hurricanes and floods.

Tsunami A very large ocean wave caused by an underwater earthquake or volcanic eruption.

Responding to disaster

Disasters may be the consequence of a natural event, or the result of human activity. They tend to occur over a short period of time and may involve many deaths and casualties. The disaster may overwhelm the health and emergency services and lead to widespread disruption of transport systems and essential services such as water and sanitation. The key to dealing with disaster situations is to have clear plans for an effective and efficient response to deal with the disaster as it happens and with the subsequent clean-up. After the initial event is over, the reconstruction and rehabilitation of communities may take months or even years. Some disaster consequences can be avoided not only through good response planning, but also by ensuring that the physical infrastructure is able to cope, such as ensuring that building codes are adhered to.

Natural disasters result from climatological factors (hurricanes and floods) or geological events (earthquakes and volcanic eruptions) and as such tend to be seen as unavoidable and largely inevitable. On the other hand, man-made (technological) disasters are perceived to be avoidable. Natural disasters therefore tend to arouse a less judgmental response from the community than man-made disasters. However, the consequences of natural disasters can be more severe than necessary due to man-made failures, for example, failure to adhere to building codes in earthquake zones, poor management of flood barriers, lack of management of disaster coordination centres or failure to implement early warning systems (Table 12.1).

Table 12.1 Perceived differences between natural and technological disasters

	Natural disasters	Technological disasters
Nature of disaster	clean; unavoidable	dirty; contaminated
Responsibility	no agent	culpable party
Objective magnitude of loss	often great	usually less
Perceived magnitude of loss	usually minimized	usually maximized
Community support for those affected	non-judgmental	highly judgmental; ambiguous

Source: Yassi et al. (2001)

Natural disasters

Climatological events (hurricanes and floods) have the most severe environmental impact and occur more frequently than geological disasters such as earthquakes, volcanic eruptions, and tsunamis. They are also more likely to increase in occurrence due to the effects of global climate change. As you might expect by now, high middle and low income countries are not equally affected by natural disasters – 95 per cent of deaths occur in low and middle income countries and the economic losses are 20 times greater than in developed countries. Floods are the most common natural disaster and the public health impacts can vary. These include the destruction of homes and displacement of communities, the spread of infectious disease, the contamination of drinking water, the release of chemicals from storage sites and the interruption of sewerage and waste disposal systems. Table 12.2 shows the main health impacts that result from natural disasters.

As you can see in Table 12.2, geological disasters are more likely to involve death and severe injury. The psychological stress caused by these disasters also tends to be immense and to compromise the ability of the community to deal with their own needs immediately after the event. Forest fires have a similar effect. Public health problems occur secondary to population movements, food scarcity and infectious disease outbreaks that occur, particularly after volcanic eruptions, floods and tsunamis. Climate-related natural disasters such as flooding tend to be more damaging to property. They are demoralizing but they are likely to be relatively common occurrences and the community knows how to respond to them in a constructive way.

Table 12.2 Health effects of natural disasters

Health effect	Earthquake	Hurricane, high wind	Volcanic eruption	Flood	Tidal wave, flash flood
Death	many	few	varies	few	many
Severe injury (requiring extensive medical care)	overwhelming	moderate	variable	few	few
Increased risk of infectious disease	a potential problem in all major disasters; probability increases with overcrowding and deteriorating sanitation				
Food scarcity	rare (may occur as a result of factors other than food shortages)	rare	common	common	common
Major population movements	rare (may occur in heavily damaged urban areas)	rare	common	common	common

Source: Moeller (1997)

Extreme weather and global climate change

Global climate change is expected to lead to an increasing number of extreme climate events (see Chapter 10). There are two categories of climate extremes to be considered:

- extremes of climatic statistical ranges, such as very low or very high temperatures
- complex events: droughts, floods, or hurricanes.

The health effects of weather-related disasters such as droughts, floods, storms and bushfires are difficult to quantify. Initial deaths or injury tolls are reported, but the delayed consequences of the disaster are often poorly reported.

The number of natural disasters is increasing. This can be attributed to a number of causes and may in part be a consequence of the better recording of events. Compared to the 1960s, there has been a tripling in the number of natural disasters in the past ten years, according to an analysis by the reinsurance company Munich Re. This is probably partly due to increasing population vulnerability rather than to an increased frequency of extreme climatic events themselves; however, increased population vulnerability is partly a result of global climate change. For example, a large number of people live in areas at increasingly high risk of flooding particularly in low and middle income countries, and these communities tend to be poorly equipped to deal with weather extremes. This has led to the huge rise in the number of people killed, injured or made homeless by natural disasters. A recent example of this is the tsunami on the 26th December 2004 when thousands lost their lives and millions had their homes and livelihoods destroyed. A description of the tsunami and its after-effects is given in the following extract from the BBC (2005).

Tsunami

On December the 26th 2004 a series of earthquakes with epicentres off the Northern Sumatra (Aceh) in Indonesia and the resultant tsunamis hit Southeast Asia causing serious damage and loss of life. The earthquake measured 9 on the Richter scale, the largest earthquake in 40 years. The initial priorities were to ensure clean water, adequate shelter, food, sanitation and healthcare for the 3–5 million people affected, and to identify and bury thousands of bodies. A week after the disaster there was widespread shortage of clean water and a risk of disease outbreaks. Health education received a high priority in India and Sri Lanka to help prevent the spread of disease. Providing health services to displaced people was a significant challenge. Six weeks after the disaster the second phase of the post-disaster health programme is in place and the focus is on rebuilding infrastructure, increasing capacity and assessing and rehabilitating their health systems. The mental health and nutritional status of many tsunami survivors remain serious concerns (WHO 2005).

The worst affected area was Aceh on the island of Sumatra in Indonesia; more than 70% of the inhabitants of some coastal villages are reported to have died. The exact number of victims will never be known, the number of homeless is estimated at 800 000. After the disaster, at least 100 aid organisations and UN agencies were operating in Indonesia. They provided emergency food, water and shelter to about 330,000 people and now are constructing temporary settlements for 150,000 families.

Indonesia was hardest hit in terms of loss of life and physical damage, but seems to have escaped the worst of the tsunami's economic disruption. The main affected area, Aceh, is rich in resources but far from crucial to overall output. The government estimates that reconstruction will cost $4.5bn (US) over the next three years.

The reconstruction bill for Sri Lanka, the second hardest hit country, is expected to be enormous because the damaged infrastructure was more developed than in many affected areas. There is expected to be a loss of valuable tourist revenue all over the region as resorts were devastated and many foreigners were killed in the disaster.

 Activity 12.1

Haiti was struck by a huge storm in September 2004 that killed more than 1,100 people, leaving many other thousands injured or homeless. Read the following article from Joseph Delva (2004) that reported the storm. Then answer the question: What are the health effects of this disaster?

 Hundreds buried in Haiti

Haiti began burying hundreds of flood victims in mass graves on Wednesday while emergency food was distributed to some of the thousands of people made homeless by Tropical Storm Jeanne.

The death toll rose to 1,008 in the Artibonate region around the northern coastal city of Gonaives and 72 in Haiti's Northwest province, said Dr. Carl Murat Cantave, a government official. Another 1,000 people were missing and the final death count was likely to hit 2,000, he said.

Walls of water roared down from the Caribbean country's deforested hills as the storm passed north of Haiti during the weekend, and left Gonaives and Port-de-Paix, another northern city, under a dense crust of mud. Government workers and U.N. peacekeepers were burying the dead in mass graves to prevent the spread of disease. Truckloads of bodies in plastic bags were delivered for burial at the Bois Marchand cemetery near Gonaives and police were called in to calm neighbors who angrily protested the mass burials, Cantave said.

The U.N.'s World Food Program said its first convoy of trucks carrying 40 metric tons of food arrived Tuesday night and aid agencies were distributing rice, beans, cooking oil and loaves of fresh bread. 'At this point we think at least 175,000 people are affected across the country. Many of them were already very vulnerable and now, they have lost their homes, their entire crops, their animals and the few belongings they had,' said the WFP country director, Guy Gauvreau. 'It is a huge disaster. The water has just washed away everything,' he said.

Police tried to keep order as desperately hungry people swarmed the food distribution sites. One policeman was hit by a rock and injured while trying to hold back the crowd. The WFP has long provided food for 500,000 people in the poorest country of the Americas, and increased operations after a violent revolt forced ex-President Jean-Bertrand Aristride to flee into exile on Feb. 29.

Devastating floods and mudslides in May, in which about 2,000 people died, further aggravated the humanitarian disaster facing the country. Haiti is chronically vulnerable to flooding because of widespread deforestation caused by Haitians digging up roots to make charcoal for cooking.

U.N. forces maintaining the peace after Aristide's departure were helping with rescue and relief efforts. The international Red Cross, meanwhile, launched a worldwide appeal for $3.3 million to help the flood victims.

Haitian-American hip-hop artist Wyclef Jean joined aid workers. 'I came here to see my people, to see their desperation and to assess the situation and see how we can help,' Jean told Reuters, 'I want to be able to tell the world about the disaster I witnessed here.' He said he was trying to organize a 'peace concert' for Haiti later this year featuring top international stars.

Jeanne also killed 11 people in the Dominican Republic, which shares the island of Hispaniola with Haiti, and two in the U.S. Caribbean territory of Puerto Rico. By 5 p.m. on Wednesday, Jeanne was 500 miles east of Great Abaco island in the northeastern Bahamas and moving slowly west-southwest. Packing winds of 100 mph, the storm was expected to swing west eventually and may threaten the east coast of the United States next week, the U.S. National Hurricane Center said. Florida has already been battered by three big hurricanes this season.

Two other storms continued to swirl through the Atlantic. Hurricane Karl was about 1,400 miles west-southwest of the Azores and unlikely to threaten land. Tropical Storm Lisa was also far from land, at about, 1,205 miles west of the Cape Verde islands.

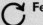 **Feedback**

Health effects

- death
- psychological effects of grief; loss of family, homes and livelihoods
- sanitation-related diseases
- lack of food and water

Other effects

- destruction of the infrastructure leading to loss of crops and food shortages; contaminated crops
- economic effects of loss of exports; loss of tourist trade; diversion of national funds for clean-up and damage relief

Floods

River floodplains have always provided sites for agricultural settlements; they are flat, fertile and the river provides a means of transport and communication. These are still important places for settlement and the communities in these areas can be quite dense. Flooding in these areas can be a result of heavy rain or a rapid snow melt. Flooding can also occur along the shores of lakes. Finally, marine coasts associated with tropical storms can experience wind-driven storm surges as well as the rain which can both cause flooding.

Floods have a benefit to the ecosystem; they leave behind nutrient-rich silt, they recharge groundwater and they refill wetlands. Human activity has contributed to the increase of flooding by removing vegetation through logging, overgrazing stock, mining, urbanization and forest fires. These all result in a more rapid run-off into streams; the resulting sediment carried into the rivers and streams makes them shallower. Floods are responsible for the highest proportion (39 per cent) of deaths from natural disasters. People living on flood plains often have no choice about where they live, particularly in low income countries. The following extract from a newspaper report by Chowdhury (2003) describes the repercussions of a flood in Bangladesh, a low-lying country with a large river delta. Wealthy regions are able to try to mitigate the effects of the floods by building barriers along river banks, preventing building in vulnerable areas and installing sophisticated flood barriers at river mouths. However, even in areas where there are flood barriers and other mechanisms such as walls or banks in place, not all floods can be prevented.

 Bangladesh flood

In July 2003 201 were reported killed and 23 million people affected due to a flood in central Bangladesh.

On July the 23rd the health directorate announced that an outbreak of water-borne disease had killed at least one person and another 1,459 from different areas were admitted in hospitals across the country.

Roads and trains were disrupted for days as roads and tracks remained underwater. Flights were suspended for more than three days. As the water levels rise families have to remain in schools and other buildings without adequate food and clean water.

The Bangladesh government, however, has begun sending relief materials for flood affected people.

Activity 12.2

The immediate effects of a flood include death, injury and property loss. After the flood waters recede, there are continued impacts on the environment and health. What are the short-, medium- and long-term health effects of floods?

Feedback

Your answer may have included the following:

- Immediate effects: death; injury; hypothermia; electrocution
- Medium-term effects: increases in gastrointestinal infections and respiratory disease; homelessness; injury occurring during clean-up operations
- Long-term effects: mental health problems

Man-made disasters

Man-made disasters also contribute to environmental damage and can cause serious health effects to local populations. They are often the results of explosions or fires. There are likely to be both direct health effects from man-made disasters such as death and injury, but also such indirect effects as dislocation of communities, environmental damage, social disruption and economic upheaval. The extract describes the accidental chemical release in Bhopal, India.

 Bhopal disaster

In 1984, an accidental release of methyl-isocyanate into the atmosphere took place at the Union Carbide plant in Bhopal in 1984. This killed 2,800 people and injured 50,000 at the time. It is now believed that over 20,000 people died from exposure to the gas since the accident, and there are 120,000 chronically ill survivors. The parent company has always downplayed the incident, trying to blame the accident on a disgruntled employee, whereas in fact, key parts of the safety equipment designed to stop the escape of the gas were not functioning or were turned off. It is alleged that the company tried to keep compensation to a minimum. Medical services in Bhopal have failed to develop a health-care service that offers sustained relief and treatment to the communities most affected.

This incident illustrated some of the problems associated with a lack of planning for disasters. It occurred in a developing country where industrial practices may not be as rigorously controlled as in developed countries. There was public housing beside the plant; the release occurred at night, making it more difficult to alert the nearby residents; there was an additional delay in warning them; there were only limited medical facilities nearby and little understanding of the toxic nature of the leak. Even after this incident, there are still weak regulations in many countries controlling the siting of potentially high-risk industries and insufficient emergency planning for the possibility of chemical disasters. Table 12.3 lists a small selection of the variety of sources and consequences of man-made disasters. Note the catastrophic effects of explosions and dam collapse, not only in terms of lives lost but also of the numbers affected. This emphasizes the need for effective planning.

Table 12.3 A selection of man-made disasters

Year	Accident type	Location	Number killed	Number injured	Number affected
1987	maritime collision	Ferry *Dona Paz* and tanker *Victor*, Philippines	4 386	0	0
1984	pesticide gas leak	Bhopal, India	2 500	100 000	300 000
1981	poison cooking oil	Madrid, Spain	340	20 000	20 000
1942	industrial accident	China	1 549	0	0
1979	dam collapse	India	1 335	0	150 000
2002	ammunition depot explosion	Nigeria	1 000	0	20 000
1983	rail accident	Hunan Province, China	600	2 000	2 000
1977	air accident	Canary Islands	562	634	634
1984	natural gas storage tank explosion	nr Mexico City, Mexico	452	4 248	708 248
1950	methyl mercury poisoning	Minamata Bay, Japan	439	1 044	1 044
1999	intoxication	Narsingdi, Bangladesh	113	0	0
1964	stadium accident	Lima, Peru	350	500	500
1988	oil rig fire	*Piper Alpha*, Scotland	167	0	0

Source: Em Dat disaster events database (extracted 20 November 2004) http://www.cred.be

Psychological effects of disasters

When we study at natural or man-made disasters we tend to dwell on the physical consequences and longer-term public health issues including psychological problems are often overlooked. However, there are important consequences, particularly for children. After a disaster, children can become fearful and suffer from separation anxiety. They may lose motivation and have poor achievement at school or act rebelliously in an attempt to once again control their environment and circumstances. Children tend to respond well to immediate mental health interventions which can help to prevent further problems.

The situation for adults is more complicated; they tend to cope well during the event, but then experience psychological problems afterwards. A small minority may be incapable of taking effective action in the crisis and, for example, may have to be forced to move away from the direct source of danger. The longer-term consequences include nightmares, the experience of uncontrollable 'reliving' of the events, a sense of detachment from others and showing no emotion. Many disaster plans now include help to deal with the psychological effects. For example, the WHO flagged this as an important component for the disaster relief plan following the South-East Asian tsunami. Within weeks there was a comprehensive strategic plan in place for Aceh in Indonesia. The plan included: assessing the mental health needs and mapping mental health activities in Aceh; the provision of guidelines for action and training of community leaders as well as the strengthening of the mental health care system, including the Aceh Psychiatric Hospital. The plan has a detailed description of necessary actions during the emergency, rehabilitation and reconstruction phases (WHO 2005).

When a disaster occurs, mutual assistance and disaster intervention programs can significantly limit the impact. In situations where international assistance is required, for instance, after an earthquake, it can be hard for communities to cope with outside help. It is a difficult situation to manage well, but in the long run may lead to an improved outcome particularly for resource-poor countries.

Emergency response and planning for disasters

While not all disasters can be predicted, many can be prepared for. This is particularly important in areas where natural events such as floods, earthquakes or hurricanes are likely to occur. Natural disasters are expected to increase in frequency and intensity as a result of global climate change, increasing the importance of good preparedness. Most areas have plans for many different types of disaster. There are two main types of emergency plan:

1 *National or regional plan* – defines responsibilities and procedures for key personnel in emergency organizations, public health and environmental departments. Includes coordination of military and civil defence organizations.
2 *Local plan* – detailed plans, comprises lists of individuals involved and their specific responsibilities. It is coordinated with the national/regional plan.

It is essential that all these plans are clear, concise, complete, flexible and dynamic to allow for changes in circumstances. It is also important that plans are implemented by a variety of individuals and do not rely on specific people who might be unavailable at the time of the incident.

Four phases of a complete plan are described by Moeller (1997):

1 *Pre-event phase (years before)*
   Requires the anticipation of accidents and disasters likely to occur; organization of personnel and services; coordination, location and inventory of supplies and equipment in both the public and private sector; review of all community and industrial facilities and their vulnerability to disaster; definition of responsibilities of all agencies and groups in establishment of lines of communication and an emergency response centre. For example, New Zealand, like many countries, has a civil defence authority responsible for drawing up plans and coordinating agencies and has temporary shelters such as schools designated as meeting points, and a range of supplies such as blankets and vehicles set aside.
2 *Warning or alerting phase (if the disaster can be predicted)*
   Advance warning is possible for some disasters, particularly for those due to natural forces such as floods, hurricanes and tornadoes. Emergency services are able to assemble, and timely, appropriate information can be provided for the

media and the public. For instance, susceptible communities may be advised to evacuate their homes if they live in the path of a flood or a fire. While the provision of early warning systems is helpful, the establishment of these systems is constrained by their high financial costs, geographical factors, institutional failures and the lack of public awareness. The effects of the South-East Asian tsunami could have been reduced if an early warning system like the one in the Pacific Region was in place. In January 2005, the UN announced that a global warning system would be established immediately. It was in place by April 2005. This aims to improve communications for natural disasters such as hurricanes and floods throughout the world and to increase international cooperation to save lives and livelihoods.

3 *Response phase*
Fire, police and ambulance services are usually the first on the scene of a disaster. Lay volunteers may also help. For example, in Australia, each state has an emergency response service, the State Emergency Service (SES), comprising volunteers and paid staff who assist in the planning for and responding to floods, severe storms, earthquakes, road accident rescue as well as in search and rescue. The SES also provides a support role to other emergency service agencies, including the Victoria Police. The SES in Victoria has more than 5,500 volunteers who are supported by 72 staff.

4 *Recovery/rehabilitation phase*
Many of the injured require immediate advice, food, water, clothing, shelter and sanitary facilities. Longer-term public health problems also need to be considered at this stage, such as rodent or insect infestations. In India, for example, the Government of Maharashtra has a department of Relief and Rehabilitation designed to deal with these issues.

Mitigation of disaster – natural events

The effects of natural disasters can be mitigated by preparation and good planning, as described in the previous section. This includes ensuring there is adequate physical infrastructure, for instance, building standards in earthquake and hurricane areas, flood stop banks along rivers and water supplies for fire fighting in rural and urban areas. The following example looks at mitigation for earthquakes in more detail.

Earthquake preparedness

The effects of earthquakes can be reduced by strict adherence to building codes and construction techniques. Emergency response preparedness and communication have also been shown to help reduce death and injury tolls. Damage to buildings, transport, gas pipelines, water supplies and waste removal must all be minimized through adherence to construction standards. In countries that are prone to earthquakes there are also public education campaigns. For example, New Zealand schools have regular 'earthquake drills' and fire drills. There are public awareness campaigns in the media to 'fix, fasten and forget' to reduce damage to property and people, and there are clear instructions in accessible places such as in libraries. In the back of the phone book delivered to every household there are instructions on how to prepare for earthquake and other disasters, including advice on how to prepare a kit containing food, water and other supplies to last for three days in an emergency.

 Activity 12.3

The path of hurricanes can be tracked for some time before they 'come to land'. This allows some time (from hours to days) to prepare for the disaster. Design a hurricane disaster preparedness plan for a tropical island in the Pacific Ocean. Refer to the example of the hurricane in Haiti described earlier in the chapter for some ideas. Divide your plan into pre-event, warning or alerting, response and rehabilitation phases.

 Feedback

1 *Pre-event phase*

- ensure that building practices adhere to standards; plan safe refuges to escape hurricane
- provide public education for hurricane mitigation
- practise the evacuation plan with the emergency services. Check, for example, that there are sufficient roads to allow communities to evacuate; safe areas for evacuation; and effective methods of communication via the media
- ensure that sufficient hospital and emergency treatment centres are available. (In a recent hurricane that hit the Pacific island of Nuie, the only hospital was destroyed.)
- ensure that sufficient food, water and temporary shelters will be available – emergency supplies may have to be flown in or be brought by sea and there could be a weather-induced delay to either of these

2 *Warning or alerting phase*

- ensure access to best available technology for forecasting of path and speed of hurricanes

3 *Response phase*

- test the emergency service response – fire, ambulance, police, civil defence authority, local council. Ensure that there is the ability to communicate even without a telephone system

4 *Recovery/rehabilitation phase*

- coordination of a clean-up plan to reduce injuries
- ensure that there are a strategy and appropriate resources to deal with ongoing psychological effects of the disaster and to provide community support
- plan for the likelihood of food scarcity if crops are destroyed. There must be ready access to alternate provisions
- plan for the possibility that water supply and sanitation may be compromised. Again, there must be ready access to alternate provisions
- housing and other buildings may need repair or replacement; ensure that there are plans and resources for the running of government and emergency services from alternative sites

Mitigation of disaster – man-made events

To prevent or reduce the effects of man-made disasters, e.g. explosions, aircraft crashes, release of toxins, there is also a need for clear, concise contingency plans. There should first be an assessment of the phenomena that might occur and the hazards associated with each of these. Procedures should be established to help mitigate these potential scenarios and response plans should be created in the event of an accident. Most countries have safety legislation covering industrial and other processes, such as Occupational Safety and Health regulations.

Health consequences of war

Wars are another form of man-made disaster. They affect thousands of people and have the potential to inflict great harm on the environment and human health. For example, in the first Gulf War in the early 1990s, war and trade sanctions led to a three-fold increase in mortality for Iraqi children under 5 years old; more than 46,900 children died between January and August 1991 (Ascherio et al. 1992). The Allied forces claimed that strategic targeting limited civilian casualties. Electricity supplies were destroyed which cut power to hospitals and water treatment facilities. Transport links were also targeted, preventing the movement of vital supplies such as food to civilian populations. Twelve years of sanctions were in place after the first Gulf War and at least 500,000 children died because of shortages of food, medicine and medical equipment, and the collapse of sanitation systems.

Indirect environmental effects of war – refugees

One consequence of war is the creation of refugees fleeing the conflict. These people become dispossessed through ethnic targeting or destruction of their homes and are subject to public health problems and hygiene in the potentially over-crowded camps and communities where they find refuge. Children of these refugee populations often miss out on schooling and health services, and psychological damage may also be associated with the loss of families and communities and the prospect of being unable to have a settled and productive life for the foreseeable future. Additional environmental damage may result from the search for food and firewood. The following extract by Capak (2001) outlines the environmental health management that should be established in refugee/displaced persons camps:

 Environmental health management in refugee camps

People who are suddenly displaced by the events of war and forced to migrate are usually not able to take their belongings with them. Such refugees are forced to depend on assistance to meet their most basic needs, such as food, shelter, medical care and water. In assessing what public health measures are appropriate, officials in refugee/displaced persons camps must consider the following: the types of makeshift shelters being used, the physical environment, the demographic profile of the people in the camp, and the extent and type of disease circulating in the population. The goal of the resulting public health measures should primarily be to prevent the occurrence and spread of diseases favoured by this situation. The process of identifying needs and setting priorities requires an immediate assessment of the population's health and nutritional status as well as a rapid environmental health assessment of the available accommodation. A monitoring and reporting system should be established to assess the effectiveness of the measures, and to ensure the timely detection of newly developed risks.

Environmental health measures include the following:

Selection of site and accommodation

- The site should be selected according to the facilities needed to provide hygienic and healthy conditions.
- Flood areas and natural foci of infection must be avoided.
- The accommodation site should afford an adequate protection against inclement weather conditions.
- Overcrowding should be avoided.

Water supply

- Ensure water is adequate in quantity and quality (consider access to water treatment and cooking facilities) and protect the source of water and water supplies from pollution.

Refuse disposal

- Build hygienic field toilets according to the planned length of stay.
- Provide waste water drainage, solid waste collection and disposal, and incineration of medical wastes.

Food wholesomeness and food hygiene

- Distribute dried and preserved foods.
- Prepare food individually.
- Place storerooms (if they exist) and community feeding facilities under health surveillance, and provide hygienic food preparation courses.

Insect and rodent control

- Controls should be based on prevention.

In addition, provisions must be made for child immunization, health education, patient treatment, drug supply, medical personnel, and a health service scheme, including a system for referrals to in-patient facilities.

Direct environmental effects of war

While the indirect effects described are serious, they affect a specific and limited population, but the environmental and health issues associated with modern weaponry are likely to be global in their impact. The damage caused by chemical, biological and nuclear weapons may lead both to the widespread distribution of serious pollution and to economic disruption internationally. Guerrilla warfare, terrorism, and deliberate sabotage also present potential threats to the immediate environment.

Chemical warfare

Chemical warfare, introduced on a large scale in World War I, involves the controlled release of toxic chemicals, usually nerve toxins or intensely irritating agents. When used in the field, these poisons are indiscriminate in their effects and may affect civilians or troops on either side, as well as wildlife or domestic animals. These agents can cause considerable local damage and may wipe out entire villages. Although chemical weapons have been outlawed since 1899 by an international agreement known as the Hague Declaration, there have been many documented instances of their use and many more suspected incidents in which absolute proof has been lacking or controversial.

Chemical weapons have been used by terrorist groups. In 1995 a terrorist group in Japan, Aum Shinrikyo, released 'sarin' (a nerve gas) on the Tokyo subway. Twelve people were killed, and over 5,000 suffered the effects of the gas.

Biological warfare

Biological warfare, which is even more difficult to regulate, involves the controlled release of pathogens such as viruses and bacteria. In the few instances in which it has been tried, there have been limited outbreaks of disease involving local residents and wildlife. The Geneva Convention has outlawed these weapons since 1925. The most recent publicized use of biological agents was a series of attacks where anthrax (a potentially fatal bacteria) was sent through the post to various targets in the USA in 2001. The attacks infected 23 people, killed 5, and caused widespread disruption as buildings were evacuated and shut down.

Nuclear warfare

The only time that nuclear weapons have been deliberately used in war was by the USA against Japan at the end of World War II. Atom bombs were dropped in 1945 on the cities of Nagasaki and Hiroshima. The consequence of that action was the death of 210,000 people by the end of the year; more died subsequently due to radiation illness and there remains a legacy of second-generation birth defects and cancers. There was also a great deal of destruction at the site of the bombs and in the surrounding areas of both cities. The testing of nuclear weapons in the South Pacific and elsewhere has had important environmental impacts and has affected the original inhabitants, who had to be moved from the area. Other issues surrounding nuclear arms include local contamination from inadequate or unsafe storage, accidental release of nuclear material and acts of terrorism.

Guerrilla warfare, terrorism and deliberate environmental destruction

Many conflicts in the twentieth century involve guerrilla warfare rather than full-scale conflict. This avoids direct engagement and relies instead on periodic ambush. The dominant force will destroy villages and the countryside, causing environmental destruction in order to flush out the guerrilla groups. For example, during the Vietnam War, 'Agent Orange' (a herbicide containing 2,4,D and 2,4,5,T, both of which contain dioxins as contaminants) was sprayed on the jungle to cause defoliation and reveal the guerrillas. It has been blamed for cancers, diabetes, and birth defects in the local populations and health problems in the US military veterans.

Similarly, landmines are a serious issue world-wide; there are 15,000–20,000 casualties each year from landmines and unexploded ordinance. Many of these are in countries that are no longer in a state of war. The widespread presence of such mines in countries such as Mozambique and Angola means that large tracts of land are unable to be used for cropping and agriculture. These countries can ill afford to lose arable land.

Ecological vandalism is another consequence of warfare. The oil-field fires started by the Iraqi Army in the Kuwait War had a limited military purpose, but caused ecological destruction and air pollution for many weeks until they were brought under control.

Until the attacks on the World Trade Center and other targets on the 11th of September 2001, the public health impact of terrorism was relatively small scale. The attacks killed 2,749 in the World Trade Center alone and injured tens of thousands; billions of dollars worth of damage was done. Terrorist attacks continue in all parts of the world. In 2003 there were 208 acts of international terrorism with 625 people killed and 3,646 injured. While the number of attacks and deaths decreased in 2003, the number injured increased as there were more attacks on 'soft' targets such as places of worship, hotels and commercial districts (US Department of State 2004). This type of attack interferes with civil society and causes stress as well as physical damage.

Summary

The environmental, health and economic costs of disasters – natural as well as man-made – are immense. In the past 20 years, three million deaths have been caused by natural disasters alone. Complex climate-related disasters are likely to increase as a result of global warming, threatening already vulnerable communities. Planning for disaster prevention and relief is essential for natural and man-made disasters. Wars and terrorism affect thousands of people both directly and indirectly and have the potential to inflict great harm on the environment and human health.

References

Ascherio A, Chase R, Cote T et al. (1992) Effect of the Gulf War on infant and child mortality in Iraq. *New England Journal of Medicine* 24; 327(13): 931–6.

BBC (2005) Update on T http://news.bbc.co.uk/1/hi/world/4126019.stm, Tuesday, 1 March, 2005.

Chowdhury SI, (2003) *The New Age*, Dhaka, 23 July: http://www.internationalflood network.org/index_e.html

Delva JG (2004) Hundreds buried in Haiti as flood deaths top 1,000. Reuters Ltd.

Moeller DW (1997) *Environmental Health*. Cambridge, MA, Harvard University Press

US Department of State (2004) Patterns of Global Terrorism 2003: http://www.state.gov/s/ct/rls/pgtrpt/2003/33771.htm

A Yassi, T Kjellstrom, T de Kok and TL Guidotti (2001) *Basic Environmental Health*. Oxford: Oxford University Press.

Further reading

Blaikie P, Cannon T, Davies I and Wisner B (2004) *At Risk* (2nd edn). London: Routledge.

Centre for Epidemiology of Disasters: http://www.cred.be

Em Dat: Centre for Epidemiology of Disasters http://www.cred.be

Handmer J (2003) Adaptive capacity: what does it mean in the concept of natural hazards? in Smith JB, Klein RTJ, and Huq S. (eds) *Climate Change and Adaptive Capacity*. London: Imperial College Press.

International campaign to ban landmines: http://www.icbl.org/

International Federation of Red Cross and Red Crescent Societies: http://www.icrc.org/

News24 (2005) http://www.news24.com/News24/World/Tsunami_Disaster/0,,2-10-1777_ 1667234,00.html, Report for 25 February 2005.

Noji E (ed) (1996) *Public Health Consequences of Disasters*. Oxford: Oxford University Press.

Pan American Health Organization disaster archive: http://www.paho.org/English/dd/Ped/ disasterarchives.htm

Regional Disaster Information Centre, Americas and the Caribbean (CRID): http:// www.crid.or.cr/crid/ing/index_ing.html

WHO (2005) http://www.who.int/hac/crises/international/asia_tsunami/en/

13 The urban environment and health

Overview

Five per cent of the world's population lived in urban areas in 1800, 15 per cent in 1900, by 2025, it is estimated that 50 per cent of the population will live in urban areas. Urbanization – the increasing concentration of people and economic activities in towns and cities – brings economies of scale and proximity to infrastructure. Services that reduce the risks of injury, illness and premature death can be considered to be beneficial for health, although in low and middle income nations, the benefits are spread unevenly. Large sections of the urban population live in tenements, boarding houses and illegal settlements where conditions are very poor and health burdens very high. In this chapter you will be looking at the environmental health issues associated with urbanization, at how they affect different populations within cities and how cities might be designed for the optimal health of their inhabitants.

Learning objectives

By the end of this chapter, you will be better able to:

- **describe the basic requirements of human settlements**
- **appreciate the scope of health problems associated with urbanization**
- **compare the differential impact of urban environmental problems on the health of different groups within cities**
- **summarize the principles of planning for a healthy city**

Key terms

Ecological footprint Measures the amount of renewable and non-renewable ecologically productive land area required to support the resource demands and absorb the wastes of a given population or specific activities.

Infrastructure The basic facilities, services and installations needed for the functioning of a community, such as transport and communication systems, water and power lines, schools, post offices and prisons.

Socioeconomic differentiation Differences between individuals depending on their standing in the community with respect to their income, wealth or educational attainment.

Urban area Geographic area often defined as having a population of 10,000–50,000 or more.

The urban environment

High income countries have tended to have the highest proportion of people living in cities although this trend is changing, especially in countries with a rapidly accelerating pace of economic growth; 90 per cent of urban growth in the next 20 years is predicted to occur in low and middle income countries. One of the consequences of this is that population influx into cities may occur at a faster rate than the infrastructural development can cope with, and new migrants may experience new health hazards both from the urban environment and from inadequately controlled health and safety conditions of employment in new industries.

Although it has been covered in the context of other environmental issues raised in the book such as outdoor air pollution and water and sanitation, urbanization affects so much of the world's population, and will increasingly affect more, that it is useful to consider an overview of the urban environment in its own right.

Defining the urban environment

The urban environment is multifaceted: each aspect of the environment influences, and is influenced, by the others. The concept of driving forces that influence health and the environment is particularly appropriate in the urban situation. You will remember that human driving forces were identified as 'those social and economic conditions that influence human activities such as industry, the provision and use of services and household consumption'. Within a rapidly urbanizing area, particularly in poor countries, these factors are often uncoordinated or, as McMichael (1993) puts it, 'Rapid urbanisation represents a profound transformation of human ecology . . . that is generally outstripping social and political responses'.

 Activity 13.1

This activity focuses on the physical, social and cultural, psychosocial, economic aspects of the urban environment. Complete Table 13.1 referring to any city that you are familiar with:

Table 13.1 Aspects of urbanization

Aspect	Example	Potential health effect	Prevention
Physical			
Social/cultural			
Psychosocial			
Economic			

1 Insert an example of one negative impact of each of the environmental influences.
2 Insert the likely health effect in each case.
3 Suggest a possible method of prevention of the negative health effect.

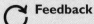

Feedback

Table 13.2 shows some examples of the answers you might have included, there are many others.

Table 13.2 Aspects of urbanization (completed)

Aspect	Example	Potential health effect	Prevention
Physical	air pollution from transport	respiratory and cardiovascular disease	reduce car numbers provide better public transport
Social/cultural	lack of education	high infant mortality	improve access to education
Psychosocial	over-crowding	mental health problems	better-quality housing
Economic	lack of employment	general health	encourage industry and services to relocate

Modifying the natural environment for urbanization

Urban areas are characterized by their high-density population, who are accommodated by the development of extensive road networks, housing schemes, service and production industries and recreational facilities. The changes in the environment that occur as a result of urbanization are shown in Table 13.3.

The largest growth in urbanization is taking place in low and middle income countries, many of which have tropical climates that exaggerate environmental changes. For example, rainfall is heavier than in non-tropical regions, causing greater problems with run-off and sedimentation. Many cities in low and middle income countries were colonial outposts that began life as small trading posts or administrative centres. Many were not in suitable sites for expansion, with

Table 13.3 Changes in the environment as a result of urbanization

Change	Effect
Water	Increased run-off
	Flood intensity increases
	Depletion of water sources
	Problem with waste water
Climate	Increased temperatures (heat island effect)
	Increased cloudiness and precipitation
	Reduced humidity, reduced wind speed
Air	Pollution increased including particulates
Ecology	Reduced vegetation and wildlife
	Introduction of exotic species
Physical	Changes of water channel
	Problem of solid waste disposal

Source: Gupta and Asher (1998)

swamps, rivers, steep slopes or otherwise unsuitable topography restricting their growth. For example, Kingston, Jamaica, is situated in an area subject to seismic disturbances and intense tropical storms; these can lead to additional environmental problems and potential disaster for the citizens (Gupta and Asher 1998).

Physical aspects of the urban environment

Physical aspects of the urban environment that have an effect upon population health include water supply and quality, sanitation provision, industrial and residential pollution, housing, infrastructure and the city's geographical situation (e.g. on a flood plain or an earthquake belt).

Road transport has two important physical influences: first, it is the major source of air pollution, and, second, motor vehicles cause accidental injuries.

Indoor air pollution can cause acute respiratory infections in children and chronic lung disease in adults. In many cities 30–60 per cent of the population live in over-crowded, poor quality housing with implications for the spread of airborne infections, and exposure to heat, cold and damp.

Social and cultural aspects of the urban environment

One of the blights of urban living has been termed socioeconomic differentiation, which points to unequal access to economic resources and differing opportunities for health according to an individual's standing in the community with respect to their income or occupation.

Living in urban centres can offer great potential gains, such as access to paid work and health-care facilities. However, in many cities, particularly in low and middle income countries, growth in urban populations is synonymous with growth of urban poverty.

An increase in the urban population due to migration and high fecundity leads to rapid urban growth beyond the service capacity of the urban governments. This creates a situation where poverty is reinforced by lack of basic housing, services and employment infrastructure. The cities undergoing most rapid growth are in poor countries and their urban fringe dwellers live in extreme deprivation. Migrants to urban areas include displaced rural workers who may be looking for paid work or in search of food and shelter, or are moving due to the deterioration of rural life secondary to over-crowding or environmental degradation. Urban migration also occurs between countries; economic migrants move from poor to richer countries.

Slums and squatter settlements represent a series of trade-offs between poor living quality and close proximity to jobs and markets and having no access to infrastructure and the informal and intermittent supply of urban services. The extract describes the rise in slum development in Mumbai, India, and the largely failed attempts to rectify the problem. Consequently, the slums and the environmental and health problems are growing at a faster rate here than for the rest of the urban population. However, living on the margins does not necessarily mean a breakdown of social organization; squatter settlements can be stable communities with strong community organization and the provision of cheap or informal labour to support the economy as the following extract by Lanegran (1999) illustrates.

 Slums in Mumbai, India

The city of Mumbai is based on the island of Bombay in the west of India and has one of the world's best natural harbours. It is India's second largest, but most modern city. Slums (*zopadpattis*) have always existed in Mumbai. When the original fort was developed, the native villages moved close to the centre as squatter settlements. There was no planning, construction of infrastructure or implementation of facilities such as water, sewage, and drainage. Over the passage of time, this has led to problems for Mumbai's poor population. Mumbai has a very dense population with 16,500 people per square mile and a scarcity of housing. Before 1950, slums were predominantly found around the mills, on the western part of the island. Health care and provisions to these areas were largely ignored. In 1954 there was a slum clearance, yet despite this, the slum population has increased and today slum dwellers make up 60 per cent of Mumbai's population, approximately seven million people.

The scarcity of housing has meant the slums have spread wherever they can find space, including onto roads. Conditions are difficult. Inhabitants have to deal with issues such as constant migration, lack of water, no sewage or solid waste facilities, lack of public transport, pollution and housing shortages. Infant mortality in these areas is as high as there are no amenities in rural India. General Hospitals in the Greater Mumbai region are over-crowded and under-resourced. There is either too little water in the area for drinking and sanitation, or in the monsoon season too much water and flooding.

There have been moves by the government to improve the slum areas. In 1985, the Slum Upgradation Project began. The aim of the project was to offer secure, long-term, legal plot tenure to slum households if they agreed to invest in their housing. The programme managed to target only the 10–12 per cent of the slum population who were capable of upgrading their homes. It offered no incentive for those without homes. Despite the attempts to remedy the slum problem of Mumbai, the slums are still growing.

Economic infrastructure

A viable economic infrastructure is vital if a city is to achieve sustainability, growth and provide a healthy environment. The provision of adequate water supplies, sewerage, lighting, housing and communications support is essential but there must also be employment available for workers with a diversity of skills. Manufacturing industries or the service-led economy may predominate. However, reliance on a narrow economic base such as shipbuilding is dangerous, because a decline in that particular industry will depress the entire city. The economic infrastructure also depends on the type of government in place at both municipal and national levels, and the policies that it advocates.

Health and the urban environment

At the beginning of the chapter you began to think about the health effects associated with different aspects of the urban environment. Table 13.4 illustrates in

Table 13.4 Specific health effects and the urban environment

Diseases	Socioeconomic environment	Physical environment	Behavioural, lifestyle
Communicable – acute respiratory infections	over-crowding – sharing accommodation to lower rent costs	air pollution; house site; ventilation; house dust; building materials; damp; heating materials	tobacco smoking; cooking and heating practice; use of health services; occupation
Communicable – diarrhoeal diseases	cost of water; education of mother; access to individual water supply	water quality; water source; excreta disposal	hygiene behaviour; weaning practice; use of health services; water storage
Non-communicable – accidents	maternal care – (working) mothers not having time to look after children crowding – constraints of space for cooking, poor access to childcare facilities for poor families	road – density of traffic; home – repair of house; cooking site; cooking materials	cooking practice, occupation, maternal care patterns, cultural practices
Psychosocial – mental distress	living in a shanty area, insecurity of tenure, migration status, insecurity of income, unemployment	quality of housing, physical security of area, child recreation facilities	lack of self-esteem (related to employment and life circumstances), migration status, cultural conflict, gender, socioeconomic frustration

detail some specific health effects and the multi-factorial environmental causes or exacerbating factors.

In low and middle income countries with rapid urbanization there are settlements on unsuitable marginal land, poor housing in settlements or shanty towns, large increases in population density, an uncontrolled increase in pollution (air, water and land) and a lack of basic infrastructure (electricity, water, sewerage, waste disposal, health care, education). These circumstances have meant a rise in these areas of communicable diseases, known as the 'diseases of poverty'. These include malaria and schistomasiasis, Chagas' disease, hookworm and a range of gastric and respiratory diseases, nutritional deficiency and drug-related illness. High-density living is also associated with over-crowding which leads to non-communicable diseases – specifically accidents in the home and on the roads.

The stresses of urban life have been linked to an increase in depression, suicide and substance abuse. It is suggested that the breakdown or lack of social relationships caused by over-crowding and migration creates a perception of loss of control which causes stress and leads to mental health problems.

Pollutants such as lead are also cited as factors related to mental impairment, particularly in children.

Health differentials within the urban environment

The lives of those who live in urban areas have been found to be generally healthier than those in rural areas. These findings do not take into account the vast wealth differential within urban areas. The rich can afford to live very well and are able to take full advantage of the city's many cultural and economic opportunities, while the urban poor may live very wretched lives – in many cases, far worse than the rural poor.

Environmental consequences of poverty in cities can broadly be described in terms of lack of access to:

• basic amenities, such as water, sanitation and waste disposal
• suitable housing and adequate living space
• habitable land.

Access to education, employment, a good diet and occupational safety are also important, and are frequently inequitably denied to the urban poor.

Urban differentials and mortality

Table 13.5 illustrates how the health of the population varies both between and within two cities: São Paulo in Brazil and Accra in Ghana. These are both cities undergoing expansion in low income countries in South America and Africa respectively.

Table 13.5 shows how the mortality rates of three diseases vary within and between cities. For circulatory diseases: São Paulo has a higher overall mortality rate; however, Accra has a larger differential). For infectious and parasitic diseases: Accra has a mortality rate approximately three times that of São Paulo. For respiratory diseases there are similar mortality rates between the two cities, but a larger differential from best to worst in Accra.

Table 13.5 Age-adjusted mortality differentials between socioenvironmental zones in São Paulo, Brazil (1992) and Accra, Ghana (1991)

Socio-economic zone	Circulatory diseases rate/10 000 (RR)		Infectious and parasitic diseases rate/10 000 (RR)		Respiratory diseases rate/10 000 (RR)	
	São Paulo	Accra	São Paulo	Accra	São Paulo	Accra
1 (Worst)	23.0	16.4	2.7	9.2	8.4	7.6
	(1.2)	(2.3)	~(1.9)	(2.0)	(1.2)	(1.9)
2	22.4	14.6	2.2	14.4	7.7	7.5
	(1.2)	(2.1)	~(1.6)	(3.0)	(1.1)	(1.9)
3	19.1	13.0	1.9	10.1	7.1	6.5
	(1.0)	(1.9)	(1.4)	(2.1)	(1.0)	(1.6)
4 (Best)	19.4	7.0	1.4	4.7	7.0	4.0
	(1.0)	(1.0)	(1.0)	(1.0)	(1.0)	(1.0)

Note: Mortality rates per 10,000 and relative risks (RR)

In both cities, the poor are more severely affected than the rich, but the disparity is greater in Accra. This is because in the early 1990s Accra was still in transition. However, the disparity between rich and poor not only occurs in cities in transition; the same gradient (although less steep) is found in high income cities such as London.

Environmental risk transition

Health transition is linked to the environment. Figure 13.1 illustrates how in poor settlements, environmental issues are local and related to sanitation and housing. These problems create increases in infectious disease rates. As settlements increase in wealth and development, the effect on the environment is less immediate and is caused by polluting emissions from vehicles and factories in particular.

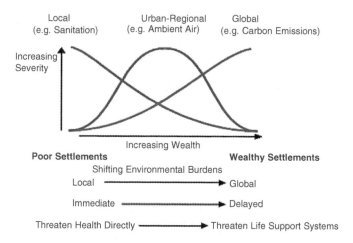

Figure 13.1 Urban environmental transition

Environmental health problems vary between cities and are related to their current stage of development. Planning for healthy cities can help to manage environmental transitions so as to affect the most beneficial outcome for the environment and for health in growing urban areas. Table 13.6 illustrates how urban environmental issues are dealt with in cities with different levels of income and how cities with high incomes have the potential to establish healthy environments.

Urbanization and sustainable development

The environmental impact of urbanization does not stop at the city walls or near the source of pollution. The wider environmental impact also needs to be considered.

Table 13.6 Urban environmental issues and development

Sector or problem area	Low	Lower-middle	Upper-middle	High
Water supply service	Low coverage, high bacteria contamination, inadequate quantity for hygiene (high risk of food contamination and infectious diseases)	Low access by poor residents and informal neighborhoods	Generally reliable, but rising demand causing shortages in resource supply	Good supply but high total consumption; some concern with trace pollutants
Sanitation	Very low coverage, open defecation in some neighborhoods and low ratio public toilets to residents; high risk of diarrheal diseases	Better coverage of latrines and public toilets, but poorly maintained; low sewerage coverage	More access to improved sanitation, but still large numbers of residents in large cities not covered especially in informal settlements; most wastewater discharge untreated	Full coverage; most wastewater treated
Drainage	Storm drains very inadequate, poorly maintained; frequent flooding, creating high risk of water-related disease vectors (mosquitoes)	Somewhat better than in low income	Better drainage; occasional flooding	Good drainage; very limited flooding
Water resources	Mixed sewerage and storm water runoff to water bodies causing bacterial pollution and silting	Risk of groundwater contamination from poorly maintained latrines and untreated sewage	Private wells drawing down groundwater; severe pollution from industrial and municipal discharge	High levels of effluent controls and treatment to reduce pollution
Solid waste management	Little organized collection; recycling by informal sector, open dumping or burning of mixed wastes; high exposure to disease vectors (rats, flies)	Moderate coverage of collection service, little separation of hazardous waste; mostly uncontrolled landfills	Better organized collection; severe problems but growing capacity for hazardous waste management; semicontrolled landfills	Increased emphasis on total waste reduction, resource recovery, and preventing hazardous waste; controlled landfills or incineration

Continued

Table 13.6 *Continued*

Sector or problem area	Low	Lower-middle	Upper-middle	High
Air pollution	Indoor and ambient air pollution from low-quality fuels for household uses and power generation	Growing ambient air pollution from industrial and vehicular emissions (high per-vehicle, due to inefficient fuels and vehicles)	Ambient air pollution still serious (but greater capacity to control especially industrial sources)	Ambient air pollution mainly from vehicles (due to high volume of vehicle kilometers)
Greenhouse gas emissions	Very low per capita	Low but growing per capita	Rapidly increasing, mainly due to motorization	Very high per capita
Land management (environmental zoning of fragile sites and prepara-tion for new settlements)	Uncontrolled land development; intense pressure from squatter settlements on open sites	Ineffective or inappropriate land-use controls, pushing new settlements toward urban periphery; continued high population growth	Some environmental zoning	Regular use of environmental zoning; little population growth, but rising incomes press for more land consumption for existing residents
Accident risk	In-home and workplace accidents due to crowding, fires	Increased risks of industrial workplace and traffic accidents (pedestrians and nonmotorized vehicles)	Transport accidents increasing, but some mitigation and emergency treatment response	Rate of industrial and transport accidents reduced despite increasing travel (vehicle kilometers)
Disaster management	Natural disasters produce massive loss of life and property especially in settlements in disaster-prone areas; little capacity for mitigation or emergency response	Somewhat better than in low-income, although with increasing risk of industrial disasters	Increasing awareness and capacity for disaster mitigation and emergency response	Good capacity for mitigation and response

Note: Cities grouped by estimated city product (city average income calculated by national accounts methods). Sample is of cities (including in OECD countries) with available data and is not statistically representative. Low income defined as city product below $750 per capita a year; lower-middle as $751–2,499; upper-middle as $2,500–9,999; high as above $10,000.
Source: World Bank (2003)

Peri-urban developments

As urban centres begin to sprawl, the development around them – known as peri-urban – begins to grow. This includes high and middle income residential dwellings, industrial estates, horticultural developments and cheap accommodation or settlements. These areas intersperse and are served by growing transport networks.

In poor countries there has been a shift to the fringes of urban centres as a result of overloaded rural economies which change the way in which the rural economy functions. Cities adversely impact upon ecosystems, directly via pollution and the use of farmland and coastal areas for urban development, and indirectly by disconnecting humans from the rhythms of nature (McMichael 1993).

Ecological footprint

There has been a recent trend to try and describe the 'footprint' of a city, namely the impact that it has on its environment. Urban areas rely on importing food, water, energy, minerals and other resources from outside their boundaries. They also produce large quantities of waste that pollute air, water and soil, inside and outside of the city limits. The land area covered by cities covers about 5 per cent of the planet, but supplying the resources for urban dwellers involves 73 per cent of the habitable land area. There are, however, some environmental benefits from urbanization. The large concentration of suitable material makes recycling economically viable. Urban dwellers generally have lower birth rates than rural dwellers and there are more opportunities to educate and mobilize residents on environmental issues. Biodiversity can potentially be preserved by protecting habitats as the population is based in a circumscribed area, although this has been balanced against the damage incurred in providing the cities with resources.

Cities can be more sustainable if re-use, recycling, waste reduction, pollution prevention and efficient use of resources are prioritised. Other initiatives such as tree planting have a number of benefits described in the following extract from two websites. There is wide scope for urban gardens, both private and communal, to provide fresh food for residents.

 Benefits of urban trees

- Trees are natural buffers to harsh weather conditions. Well forested lands are consistently at least 2 to 4 degrees cooler during the summer and 1 to 2 degrees warmer during the winter than deforested land. This temperature reduction can significantly lower smog production . . . City trees also help to counter the urban heat island effect.
- Just three well-placed trees around a home can lower air conditioning bills by up to 50%, and windbreak trees can reduce winter heating bills by up to 30%.
- Tree root systems hold soil in place, preventing erosion. A city's urban forest can reduce peak storm runoff by 10 to 20%.
- Trees help cleanse the environment. During photosynthesis, trees absorb, or sequester carbon dioxide. One acre of trees provides enough oxygen for 18 people, and absorbs as much carbon dioxide as a car produces in 26,000 miles. Trees also remove sulphur dioxide and nitrogen oxide from the air.
- Trees reduce noise pollution by acting as a buffer and absorbing urban noise.

- Trees increase economic stability by attracting and keeping businesses and shoppers in a community. Mature trees also raise property values by up to 20%, according to the American Forestry Association.
- Trees help create relaxation and well-being. They relieve psychological stresses.
- A study of public housing residents in Chicago has shown that trees can play an important role in reducing urban violence.

Planning for a healthy city

The WHO is committed to a long-term initiative (WHO 1999) aimed at improving the health and well-being of those who live and work in cities. If cities are to grow and prosper in a sustainable way, they will have to:

- reduce inequalities in health status and the determinants of health
- develop public policies at the local level to create physical and social environments that support health
- strengthen community action for health
- help people develop new skills for health compatible with these approaches
- reorient health services in accordance with policy.

The WHO programme has five main themes based on successful working practice aimed at tackling some of the most serious health problems facing urban dwellers. These are:

1 Building healthy cities.
2 Addressing emerging and re-emerging diseases.
3 Addressing environmental pollution and health (with a special focus on lead and on water and sanitation).
4 Addressing child health.
5 Women's health (with a special focus on reproductive health).

The 'Healthy Cities' initiative requires the cooperation of many agencies and the underlying rationale is that it should be underpinned by the wishes of the residents of the city or town. The Healthy Cities Programme is described in the extract by Satterthwaite (1999).

 ### Cities built from the bottom up

All cities are the result of an enormous range of investments of capital, expertise and time by individuals, households, communities, voluntary organisations and non-governmental organisations (NGOs) as well as by private enterprises, investors and government agencies. Yet until recently, in many countries, city problems were assumed to be the responsibility of nations or provincial/state agencies . . . City authorities have a particularly crucial role – not only in investment, planning and management but also in encouraging and supporting the initiatives and innovations of the other groups within their city. In most cities in the South, city and municipal authorities have limited power and resources, and limited capacity to raise revenues. Although decentralisation programmes in many countries are permitting them a greater role, their effectiveness in promoting health and preventing or curing disease still depends on their skills in working with the resources and skills of other groups in the city.

A second crucial change since Habitat I in 1976 is the recognition by city authorities that a person's health can be as much the result of conditions in the home, at school or at work as the quality of health care available to them. Healthy cities need commitment and action to health promotion and disease or accident prevention with all sectors, not just from medical professionals.

. . . The core of WHO's Healthy Cities programme is to support city and municipal authorities in working with NGOs, community organisations and other groups within each city to identify and act on the most serious health and environmental problems . . . The Healthy Cities programme is not a blueprint that is given to city authorities that they have to follow but a process that permits the main health problems in a city and their causes to be identified and responses developed by all key actors within a city . . . It promotes co-operation between sectors and between different interest groups. The Healthy Cities programme supports two aspects of governance at the local level:

a) technical aspects, involving local level resource mobilisation, plan formulation, tech-nology application and resource allocation; and
b) representational and participatory aspects, including participation, channels for popu-lar representation and increased transparency and accountability in the workings of local authorities.

. . . The consultation process with the community and many different agencies and groups seeks to develop a 'vision' of the future directions of the city and to understand its current (and past) strengths and weaknesses . . .

The 'healthy cities week' in the city of Kuching in Malaysia provides an example of the wide-ranging consultation process. Questionnaires were circulated widely, asking people to list the five things they hated most and liked most in their city and wished for most. Other healthy cities programmes have used similar consultation processes, including school programmes which involved children in identifying the positive and negative aspects of the city and how the negative aspects could be tackled. The healthy city consultation process usually leads to a long-range city health plan in which priorities are set and actions of different groups and sectors are integrated.

Many healthy city programmes include the setting up of special task forces to address particularly pressing problems. Task forces are generally city-wide and are based on:

• specific settings (e.g. healthy schools, food markets, housing, settlements or neigh-bourhoods, industries) and
• specific issues such as safety, women's health, water and sanitation, priority diseases (for instance, malaria or HIV) or improved health clinics.

Activity 13.2

Read the following extract by Satterthwaite (1999) on examples of the Healthy Cities programme from quite different cities. As you read, note the similarities and differences in the programmes. What do you think makes them likely to succeed?

Examples of Healthy City programmes

Nabuel (Tunisia): This is a small city some 80 miles south of Tunis with international tourism and a ceramics industry as the main economic bases. Great efforts have been made to improve sewerage, drainage and waste disposal. A Healthy Cities project also initiated a programme to control emissions of toxic chemicals and reduce air pollution from the ceramic industry by relocating some workshops, changing the technologies used and improving the management of liquid and solid wastes. Air pollution was reduced through the use of cleaner fuel and improvements in traditional ovens. The city also organised the collection and safe disposal of medical wastes.

Glasgow (Scotland): The largest city in Scotland and also its commercial and industrial centre with a poor health record, linked partly to the city's economic difficulties and its decline as a centre of shipbuilding and heavy industry. Its Healthy Cities project recognised that health problems were not going to be solved by a medical approach, since people's health was influenced by their personal behaviour, access to services, the quality of their homes (and the costs of keeping warm) and the quality of their employment and the social and physical environments. Many local initiatives have promoted health for all, especially through community health workers.

Chittagong (Bangladesh): The second largest city in Bangladesh with around two million inhabitants; the provision of services has not kept pace with the city's rapid growth and expansion in recent decades. The Healthy City project is guided by a steering committee chaired by the mayor and including representatives from different sectors and groups. This is supported by a project office within the city corporation, zonal task forces for specific plans and actions in particular areas (for instance, one of Chittagong's 41 wards has developed a pilot 'healthy ward' programme) and sectoral task forces responsible for specific plans and actions in, for instance, housing, water and sanitation.

Feedback

The WHO initiative for Healthy Cities has shown the need for multi-sectoral co-operation for urban development projects. Attention needs to be paid to the quality of individual neighbourhoods as well as to service provisions within the city as a whole; the ability to buy adequate and safe food, to find a job, to gain education as well as access to health and other services are all as important as the availability of decent housing.

Summary

In this chapter you considered the different dimensions of urbanization, including physical social and economic aspects. You also looked at the health problems associated with rapid urbanization and at differences in health outcomes between cities in high, middle and low income countries. Finally, you considered the WHO recommendations for planning healthy cities.

References

Amokwandoh E (1992) Personal communication to Carolyn Stephens, Accra, Ghana.
Gupta A and Asher M (1998) *Environment and the Developing World: Principles, Policies and Management*. Chichester: John Wiley & Sons Ltd.

McGranahan G, Jacobi P, Songsore J, Surjadi C and Kjellén M (2001) *The Citizens at Risk: From Urban Sanitation to Sustainable Cities*. London: Earthscan Publications.

McMichael AJ (1993) *Planetary Overload: Global Environmental Change and the Health of the Human Species*. Cambridge: Cambridge University Press.

Satterthwaite D (ed) (1999) *The Earthscan Reader in Sustainable Cities*. London: Earthscan Publications.

WHO (1999) Creating healthy cities in the 21st Century, in Satterthwaite D (ed) *The Earthscan Reader on Sustainable Cities*. London: Earthscan Publications, 137–72.

World Bank (2003) *World Development Report 2003: Sustainable Development in a Dynamic World*. Washington, DC: World Bank.

Further reading

Hardoy J E, Mitlin D and Satterthwaite D (2001) *Environmental Problems in an Urbanizing World: Finding Solutions for Cities in Africa, Asia and Latin America*. London: Earthscan Publications.

Lanegran D (1999) Geography of World Urbanization course: http://www.macalester.edu/courses/geog61/espencer/slums.html

Livelihoods Connect: creating sustainable livelihoods to eliminate poverty: http://www.livelihoods.org/

McGranahan G, Satterthwaite D and Tacoli C (2004) *Urban-rural change, boundary problems and environmental burdens*. International Institute for Environment and Development (IIED): http://www.livelihoods.org/hot_topics/docs/UR_environment.pdf

Montgomery MR., Stren R, Cohen B and Reed HE (eds) (2003) *Cities Transformed: Demographic Change and its Implications in the Developing World*. Washington, DC: National Academy Press.

UN-HABITAT United Nations Human Settlements Programme: www.unhabitat.org/

14 Action at global and local levels

Overview

This book has been concerned with the relationship between the environment, health and sustainable development. Action to protect the environment comes from local, national and international levels. Grassroots movements can affect policy and also have a direct effect on health and the environment. International policy making can also influence the environment and health. This chapter explores some Local Agenda 21 initiatives and looks at whether it will be possible to live sustainably in the future.

Learning objectives

By the end of this chapter, you will be better able to:

- **distinguish between top-down and bottom-up approaches to environmental control**
- **demonstrate the need for balancing international environmental concerns with local needs and conditions**
- **give examples of the implementation of the Agenda 21 principle: 'think globally, act locally'**
- **discuss how environmental health problems can be tackled by preventive planning**

Key terms

Environmental justice The fair treatment and meaningful involvement of all people, regardless of race, ethnicity, income, national origin or educational level.

Inter-sectoral cooperation Partnerships with a variety of agencies such as local authorities, non-governmental organizations and UN bodies.

Integrating policy for environmental health and sustainable development

There are two routes to developing and initiating policies intended to tackle health problems related to environmental conditions and to achieve sustainable development. The first is the top-down approach – determining policy on a national and global scale, which then trickles down to be incorporated into local initiatives. An example of this might be to reduce ozone-depleting chemicals. The other route is a bottom-up or grassroots approach; policies arising from local needs. Grassroots policy relies on local individuals or groups coming together to express their concerns for a change in policy or action on environmental health in their area. The repercussions of such actions can end up as national policy, or remain as local initiatives, for instance, a community association lobbying for better housing conditions, or a clean water supply. The multiplication of such local initiatives can also have an effect on the global environment.

Setting environmental standards globally

While some useful legislation has been enacted at local and national levels, there is still a need for global standards for environmental health. As you have seen throughout this book, there is an increasing disparity between environmental standards in high income countries compared to those in low income countries. Transnational and multinational corporations must adhere to strict environmental and health standards in the United States or the European Union, but some corporations attempt to keep their costs low by setting up factories in low income countries and by encouraging local governments to keep their industrial standards as low as possible.

This indicates the need for trans-global environmental standards. In any discussion of global standards, the concepts of equity and environmental justice are crucial, for it is clearly unjust that the wealthier countries are able to transfer their environmental problems to the poorer countries.

Raising awareness and acting on environmental issues are difficult at the local and national level. Internationally there has been an acceptance that environmental problems need to be addressed; however, there are currently no sanctions against countries that fail to adhere to agreed environmental standards.

Environmental justice

One principle closely aligned to sustainable development that has not been specifically discussed so far is environmental justice. As defined by the US Environmental Protection Agency (EPA) in 1998:

[E]nvironmental justice is the fair treatment and meaningful involvement of all people regardless of race, ethnicity, income, national origin or educational level with respect to the development, implementation, and enforcement of environmental laws, regulations, and policies. Fair treatment means that no population, due to policy or economic disempowerment, is forced to bear a disproportionate burden of the negative human health or environmental impacts of pollution or other environmental consequences resulting from industrial, municipal, and commercial operations or the execution of federal, state, local and tribal programs and policies.

From global to local standards

Set against the global context are issues concerned with local priority setting, the local economic context and standard-setting. The local community may believe that economic and employment issues are more important to them than any safety or environmental concerns highlighted in international standards. In this instance, whose opinion carries the most weight? The benefits of providing jobs in an area and greatly increasing health outcomes and general well-being need to be set against the ill-effects of pollution and other occupational hazards. This trade-off between job security and environmental standards is a much debated area. It can be argued that the empowerment of and participation by local communities in policy making are in fact the most important issues; local people should be able to make informed choices about accepting lower environmental standards in return for economic growth and jobs which they might not enjoy if standards were higher.

National policy

Much environmental health policy is decided at a national level. National governments stand between local and global policy initiatives and are often responsible for putting policy into law. It is at the national level that strategies and actions can be initiated or maintained for good environmental health, sustained by the two principles of equity and participation, which drive them forward and help to ensure their effectiveness. There are a number of ways in which national governments can drive forward an environmental agenda that includes economic incentives, although these have mixed success. National subsidies for encouraging agriculture and industry to adopt environmentally friendly procedures have often had adverse effects, and green taxes, though effective, need to be balanced elsewhere with tax compensations.

Many countries have risen to the challenge of improving environment and health through sustainable development. They have taken steps to draw together the appropriate agencies to cooperate on reaching goals that raise the profile of health on the national agenda and improve the health of the population.

International policy making

With increasing public concern about global climate change and the powers of multinational corporations in trade negotiations, the relevance of global decision making and standard-setting becomes particularly significant. Persuading countries to agree to policy and abide by standards is often difficult, but it is essential if an impact is to be made on environmental health through the promotion of sustainable development. There are a range of international agreements supported by a variety of UN agencies, including the Millennium Declaration, the Kyoto Protocol (Agreement on Climate Change), the Basel Convention (transboundary transportation of hazardous waste), agreements on the use of ozone-depleting chemicals, and biodiversity. A great many activities by a number of different UN organizations have been undertaken to develop and sustain workable policies directed at environment, health and sustainable development. It is an important principle of

Agenda 21 that the various agencies, both UN and other, do not work in isolation but cooperate in inter-sector collaboration for the most effective responses.

It is beyond the scope of this book to go into detail on any of the accords or agreements, but one that covers health, environment and sustainable development is looked at in some more detail as an example of the complexity of drafting and implementing international agreements.

Environmental Impact assessments and human health

International initiatives to bring health, environment and sustainable development together in planning and project design are the result of the collaborations that have occurred since the Rio conference. Environmental impact assessments (EIA) for plans and projects rarely placed an emphasis on health impacts and focused instead on the impacts on the physical and biological environment. The Protocol on Strategic Environmental Assessment (the SEA Protocol) attempts to redress this imbalance by placing a special emphasis on human health, reflecting the Declaration of the Third Ministerial Conference on Environment and Health, London, 16–18 June 1999 (London Declaration on Action in Partnership: UNECE 2003). A general definition of Strategic Environmental Assessment is the formalized, systematic and comprehensive process of evaluating the environmental impacts of a policy, plan or programme and its alternatives, including the preparation of a written report on the findings of that evaluation, and using the findings in publicly accountable decision making (Thérivel et al. 1992).

SEA allows the identification and prevention of possible environmental impact at the outset of planning and programme design at the decision-making stage. An example of this might be to develop a more sustainable transport policy rather than just minimizing the environmental impact of building a road, the traditional place of environmental impact assessment. It also enables the environmental objectives to be considered on a par with socioeconomic ones, allowing better integration of sustainable development.

The aim of this protocol is to provide for a high level of protection of the environment, including health, by:

- ensuring that environmental considerations, including health, are thoroughly taken into account in the development of plans and programmes
- contributing to the consideration of environmental and health concerns in the elaboration of policies and legislation
- establishing clear, transparent and effective procedures for strategic environmental assessment
- providing for public participation in strategic environmental assessment
- these mean integrating environmental and health concerns into measures and instruments designed to further sustainable development.

There is a special emphasis on health throughout the protocol. The protocol is aimed primarily at plans and programmes that might impact on the environment, although it may also be applied to policies and legislation. The protocol defines procedures that need to be followed and it places a special emphasis on public participation, as well as on consultation of authorities. The aim of the protocol is to

fully integrate environmental objectives into plans and programmes with the aim
of furthering sustainable development.

 Activity 14.1

You are a public health representative on a committee set up to ensure a strategic
environmental assessment is carried out on a programme for creating a series of micro-
dams projects in your area. The affected area is currently agricultural land and pristine
forest; the dam will provide electricity, be stocked with fish and water will be channelled
for irrigation downstream. What will you need to include in your report?

 Feedback

These are some of the issues you would have brought before the committee.

1 The environmental and health consequences. The advantages include: provision
of electricity, irrigation, local jobs, and flood control. The disadvantages include: loss
of agricultural land, environmental and health issues associated with construction
including transport of material to site, loss of biodiversity with loss of forest, risk of
disaster if dam collapsed, water restriction to communities downstream, risk of water
and vector-borne diseases.

2 Clear, transparent and effective procedures for strategic environmental assessment
should be established and monitored.

3 Public participation should occur, i.e. all communities affected need to be fairly
consulted, including those communities living downstream of the proposed dams.

4 Sustainable development should be considered i.e. does this project meet the needs
of the current local population without jeopardizing others?

Agenda 21

If it is possible to achieve sustainable development, it is agreed that it must take
place first at the local level in order to create the groundswell of pressure needed
for global action. Local Agenda 21 is a product of the first environment
conference in Rio in 1992 and is concerned with the integration of environmental
and developmental concerns in decision making. To do this it relies on the
cooperation of government (at all levels), non-governmental agencies (e.g. health,
industry, education, charities, etc.) and local communities. One of the most
important precepts of Agenda 21 is the involvement of local representatives in
initiating and implementing regional policies that will promote development
while maintaining a healthy environment.

To achieve the aim of working co-operatively, Agenda 21 sets out four elements to
be taken into account when planning new programmes or projects:

• identify and assess health hazards associated with environment and
  development

- develop an environmental health policy incorporating principles and strategies for all sectors involved in development
- communicate and advocate this policy to all levels of society
- adopt a participatory approach to implementing health and environment programmes.

Putting ideas into action

The international community supports Agenda 21, but how well does it work in practice? There are a number of ongoing activities related to the achievement of Agenda 21 objectives throughout the world, such as the WHO Healthy Cities movement and the Sustainable Cities movement (UNCHS). The idea of inter-sector collaboration was exciting in theory, but putting theories into practice in the 1980s proved more difficult. A number of projects failed, but there were also successes and the identification of what works and what doesn't has improved. There is no single solution to each problem; for example, pit latrines may work well in one area but not another area for any number of reasons related to the environment, culture, politics health and community preferences.

Healthy Cities and Healthy Villages

You have already seen the variety of projects in the Healthy Cities programme in Chapter 13 on urbanization. You might like to look back at these examples and compare them with the Healthy Village and Island examples that follow.

The Healthy Village Programme targets rural areas with specific resources to allow communities to source the help they need to set up their own programme if there is not already one in existence. Jordon and Iran have active programmes. Water, sanitation and hygiene are often the initial focus of these projects. Local Agenda 21 promotes the importance of community involvement and this is crucial at the village level. The extract from the WHO (2003) describes how to involve communities in Healthy Village Projects.

 The role of local community committees in Healthy Villages programmes

Each village and community participating in a Healthy Villages programme should establish a committee at the local level. Local committees are essential for broad approaches to health improvement that involve a wide range of activities and individuals . . . A committee can coordinate and support the different activities and provide leadership for the community, and can serve as the community contact point with local and national government staff involved in the Healthy Villages programme. Local committees can also facilitate broad community participation in the programme, something that may be difficult to achieve by outsiders. Local committees are therefore crucial for promoting the Healthy Villages approach in a community.

Composition of a Healthy Villages committee

The composition of a local committee is critical for a successful outcome. Committee members should be influential people within the community who are respected and who are able to represent the interests of all the different community sections. If the committee reflects the narrow interests of only a small group of people, confidence may be lost in the entire programme, leading to failure. Ideally, the composition of the committee should reflect the gender balance of the community. While it may not be possible to have completely equal gender representation because of cultural and social norms, women should be adequately represented to ensure that their concerns are taken into account and dealt with sensitively. It is also helpful if staff from the national or local government are members of the committee.

The importance of local committees in Healthy Villages programmes

Local village councils in the Islamic Republic of Iran have played key roles in the successful implementation of integrated rural development programmes. The strong role played by the local committees, supported with a legal mandate, has helped rural development programmes meet the demands of the local populations and deliver sustained improvements in public health. The influential members of a community are not necessarily the people with administrative responsibilities within the community. They can also be people who are respected and act as opinion leaders, such as village chiefs, teachers, religious leaders and ordinary community members. It is best that committee members are elected by the community and have limited terms of office, to ensure that serving on the committee does not become a burden to key community members, or become a way for individuals to use the committee for personal gain. As the committee is expected to be the principal implementing body for the Healthy Villages programme, members must also have time to allocate to the committee and other Healthy Villages activities. They will also need to be accessible both to the community and to staff from local government and other bodies that provide support to the Healthy Villages programme.

 Activity 14.2

The Solomon Islands Healthy Islands project is summarized in the following extract from WHO. The project was concerned with malaria control. What other outcomes were achieved?

 Solomon Islands – Healthy Islands Project

Honiara, the . . . capital of the Solomon Islands has been christened the 'Malaria Capital of the Pacific'. During 1992 the number of reported malaria cases exceeded the total population number. In 1995, the community joined forces with WHO's Malaria Control Programme to mount an intensive effort to reduce malaria to a point where it would no longer be a public health burden. With input from international donor partners, WHO created a package of targeted control measures that covered the entire population. Diagnosis and treatment control facilities were upgraded, insecticide-treated bed nets were distributed to households (particularly for pregnant women and infants), and measures to eliminate breeding sites put into place. The construction of a special pipeline at the mouth of the river that flows through the centre of Honiara enabled water to flow constantly between the river and the sea. Together with regular cleaning of the river banks, this resulted in virtual elimination of the mosquito problem.

This activity also stimulated interest in the cleaning up the river. Improvement of sanitation and solid waste disposal in settlement areas along the river has now occurred; in areas where latrines once overhung the river, pour flush toilets have been installed, collection of household waste has been improved, and a project designed to drain a swamp along the river.

Malaria control efforts have been accompanied by an intensive community education programme that increased community awareness about malaria and what could be done to control the disease. These efforts succeeded in reducing malaria in most parts of Honiara by 74%. Moreover, for the first time, the residents of the settlement areas and the capital have seen that, together, they can act to improve their health status.

↻ Feedback

Here is an example of how a project can have additional benefits for communities and individuals over and above its initial aims. The Solomon Islands project started out with a specific target – to reduce malaria. In achieving that aim, the project also provided improved sanitation and waste removal as a by-product of insect eradication. This conferred additional benefit to the community – a better environment and individual health benefit, both lower malarial illness and fewer sanitation-related diseases. The community also benefited from working together and from the education programme associated with the programme.

A sustainable future for all?

Throughout the book you have read how human activity has impacted heavily on the planet's ecosystem. If a sustainable future for all is to be achieved, there needs to be management of natural and social environments.

In Chapter 2 (Table 2.1) the Millennium Goals were introduced; they are listed again to remind you. The UN has committed to achieving these goals by 2015. If they do so, then the world is working toward development that is sustainable and improving environment and health. They cannot be achieved without the full support of the rich nations through debt relief and technical support.

Millennium Goals

Goal 1   Eradicate extreme poverty and hunger.
Goal 2   Achieve universal primary education.
Goal 3   Promote gender equality and empower women.
Goal 4   Reduce child mortality.
Goal 5   Improve maternal health.
Goal 6   Combat HIV/AIDS, malaria and other diseases.
Goal 7   Ensure environmental sustainability.
Goal 8   Develop a global partnership for development.

It is now recognized that increasing consumption of the world's resources is unsustainable if it leads to pollution and destruction of ecosystems. The carrying capacity of the Earth depends on food production, availability of fresh water, energy supplies and biodiversity (McMichael 2001). Current patterns of consumption show that many people consume very little, whereas a very few consume a great deal. If the many consumed at the same level as the few, the Earth would not be able to supply nearly enough resources. There are also increasingly urgent issues concerning the environmental security of food and water (and other resources) that need to be addressed.

Different perspectives

The human-centred perspective includes the notion that humans are the most important part of the ecosystem and that we can control and manage nature for our benefit. An alternative way of looking at the environment is 'holistic' or 'Earth-centred'. This perspective includes the belief that we need to preserve ecosystems, limit our actions so that we do not degrade or destroy the life support systems of the Earth (and ourselves), and recognize that not all forms of economic growth are beneficial.

Attention has turned to factors that influence human activity – those driving forces introduced at the beginning of the book. The population is still increasing, fertility rates are falling, life expectancy is increasing, patterns of disease are changing from traditional (mainly infectious) to modern (lifestyle-related) diseases – such as obesity and cancer. To find a sustainable way of living we need to change our habits and patterns, we need to achieve lower population growth and consume less. The social environment and the principles of equity and environmental justice are based on the desire to reduce the divide between rich and poor. Alleviating poverty helps to preserve the environment and improve health as outlined in the Millennium Goals.

It has been argued that the precautionary principle should be applied to Earth now. This would mean that if there is good justification to assume that a given technology or process will harm the ecosystem or human health, it is important to avoid that technology or process in favour of less damaging alternatives, rather than to wait for irrefutable scientific proof before taking action.

Summary

In this chapter you have read how health, environment and sustainable development inform local, national and global policy. There are difficulties in achieving international consensus over the setting of standards relating to the achievement of sustainable development. National policy making and action also play a role in ensuring the minimizing of environmental damage and the maximizing of health benefits. The concept of environmental justice has informed the principles of Agenda 21, and its promotion of community-based enterprises directed at improving local health and environments.

References

EPA (1998) www.epa.gov/compliance/environmentaljustice/index.html Accessed 30 August 2005.

McMichael AJ (2001) *Human Frontiers, Environment and Disease*. Cambridge: Cambridge University Press.

Thérivel R, Wilson E, Thompson S, Heaney D and Pritchard D (1992) *Strategic Environmental Assessment*. London: Earthscan Publications.

UN (1993) *Agenda 21: The United Nations Plan of Action from Rio*. New York: United Nations.

UNECE (2003) SEA Protocol: http://www.unece.org/env/eia

WHO (2003) *Healthy Villages: A Guide for Communities and Community Health Workers*. Geneva: WHO.

Further reading

National sustainable development plan (UK): http://www.sustainable-development.gov.uk/

United Nations Division for sustainable development: http://www.un.org/esa/agenda21/

Glossary

Acidic precipitation Acidic chemicals dissolved in rainwater and other precipitations.

Attributable risk function The proportion of disease among the exposed that is attributable to the exposure.

Best Practical Environmental Option (BPEO) Identifies the preferred waste route in order to minimize harm and ensure the protection of the environment.

Bias Any error that results in a systematic deviation from the estimation of the allocation between exposure and outcome.

Biodiversity Variability among living organisms including the variability within and between species and within and between ecosystems.

Biomass fuel Animal dung, wood or crop residues.

Climate change A statistically significant variation in either the mean state of the climate or in its measurable variability, persisting for an extended period (typically decades or longer).

Climatological factors Climates and their phenomena including temperature, windspeed, cloud cover, hurricanes and floods.

Confounding Situation in which an estimate of the association between a risk factor (exposure) and outcome is disturbed because of the association of the exposure with another risk factor (a confounding variable) for the outcome under study.

Driving forces Factors that create the circumstances in which environmental health conditions develop or are diverted.

Ecological footprint Measures the amount of renewable and non-renewable eco-logically productive land area required to support the resource demands and absorb the wastes of a given population or specific activities.

Ecology The scientific study of the relationship between organisms and their environment.

Ecosystem A functioning, interacting system of living organisms in relation to their physical, chemical and biological environment.

El Niño A warming of the ocean surface off the western coast of South America that occurs every four to twelve years.

Environment Physical, biological, social and cultural conditions affecting people's lives and the growth of plants and animals.

Environmental justice The fair treatment and meaningful involvement of all people, regardless of race, ethnicity, income, national origin or educational level.

Equitable development Development that is based upon the principles of equity.

Equity Fairness, defined in terms of equality of opportunity, provision, use or outcome.

Eutrophication The enrichment of an ecosystem by plant nutrients, leading to possible new species change, decreased biodiversity, and toxicity.

Exposure The degree to which a person is subject to a given risk factor.

Forcing agents Any phenomenon that forces the climate to change, either natural (sunlight intensity) or man-made (pollution).

Geographic Information System (GIS) An information system used to store, view, and analyse geographical information.

Greenhouse gas emissions Gases partially or wholly produced by human activity – carbon dioxide, methane, nitrogen oxides and chlorofluorocarbons (CFCs).

Hazard A factor or exposure that may adversely affect health.

Health State of physical, mental and social well-being and not merely the absence of disease or infirmity.

Industrial revolution The use of new sources of energy from fossil fuels and the employment of new technology in the development of manufacturing industry and agricultural production.

Infrastructure The basic facilities, services and installations needed for the functioning of a community, such as transport and communication systems, water and power lines, schools, post offices and prisons.

Inter-sectoral cooperation Partnerships with a variety of agencies such as local authorities, non-governmental organizations and UN bodies.

Landfill Method of solid waste disposal in which refuse is buried between layers of soil, or the site used for such disposal.

Particulates Particulate matter, aerosols or fine particles are tiny particles of solid or liquid suspended in the air.

Patient characteristics Characteristics either inherited (e.g. a blood group), or behavioural (e.g. smoking and diet habits) or environmental factors (e.g. exposure to asbestos), associated with an increased or decreased probability (risk) of developing a disease (or other outcome).

Peri-urban On the urban margins.

Photochemical smog The reaction of hydrocarbons, for example, gasoline or methane, with nitrous oxide gases in sunlight that may lead to reduced visibility.

Precautionary principle A principle that advocates the use of prudent social policy in the absence of empirical evidence in an attempt to solve a problem.

Primary pollutant A chemical added directly to the atmosphere from natural or human activity.

Radionuclide Nuclide (an atom that exists for a measurable length of time) that decays, producing radioactive particles or rays. Radionuclides may be natural or synthetically produced.

Relative risk Estimate of the magnitude of an association between exposure and disease and indicates the likelihood of developing the disease in those exposed relative to those unexposed.

Remote sensing The measurement or acquisition of information from a distance, for example, the use of satellite images to study changes in waterways.

Risk The probability that an event will occur.

Risk transition The process by which societies move from exposure to traditional hazards to exposure to modern hazards.

Secondary pollutant A chemical formed in the atmosphere when primary pollutants react with air, chemicals or sunlight.

Sievert (Sv) A unit equivalent dose of radiation which relates the absorbed dose in human tissue to the effective biological damage of the radiation. A milisievert (mSv) is one thousandth of a sievert.

Smog A mixture of smoke and fog.

Socioeconomic differentiation Differences between individuals depending on their standing in the community with respect to their income, wealth or educational attainment.

Stratospheric ozone depletion Reduction of ozone in the stratosphere.

Sustainable development Meeting the needs of the present generation without compromising the ability of future generations to meet their needs.

Tsunami A very large ocean wave caused by an underwater earthquake or volcanic eruption.

Ultraviolet (UV) radiation Invisible electromagnetic radiation from sunlight.

Urban area Geographic area often defined as having a population of 10,000–50,000 or more.

Vector An organism, such as an insect, that transmits a pathogen from one host to another.

Waste hierarchy Methods of waste disposal from re-use (best environmental option) to disposal (worst).

Water-based disease Caused by disease-causing agents that spend part of their life cycle inside an intermediate aquatic host.

Water-borne disease Caused by the transmission of disease in drinking water.

Water-related vector-borne diseases Diseases spread by insects that either breed in water, or are found nearby.

Water-washed Diseases which could be prevented through provision of increased quantities of water.

Water scarcity Not enough water to supply all users' needs.

Index

AAMA, 53
accidents
  fatal workplace accidents, 46–9
  traffic, 4, 54
  urban environment, 188, 192
accommodation strategy, 148
Accra, Ghana, 189–90
acidic precipitation, 159, 209
acute health effects, 112
acute respiratory disease, 7, 188
Africa
  model of malaria distribution, 147
  Sub-Saharan Africa, 94
  see also under individual countries
Agenda 21, 20, 200–1, 202–5
Agent Orange, 180
Ahern, M., 63
aid, 22, 174–5
air pollution see indoor air pollution; outdoor air pollution
air quality, 114–18, 140
  concepts and standards, 115–17
  management of in low and middle income countries, 118
  setting standards, 114–15
alerting/warning phase, 175–6, 177
Alkali Act 1863, 18
aluminium, 159
ammonia, 116
Angola, 181
animals, 158–9
Anopheles mosquitoes, 94–6
anthrax, 180
APHEA-2 study, 112
arsenic, 100, 101, 102
artemisinin, 162
asbestos, 125
Ascherio, A., 178
ash, 83
Asher, M., 18, 59–60, 164, 165, 185, 186
Asia, 71, 73, 94

South-East Asian tsunami, 167, 169–70, 174–5, 176
  see also under individual countries
association, 133
asthma, 129
attributable risk fractions, 130, 209
Aum Shinrikyo, 180
Australia, 47, 49, 151
  emergency response services, 176
  preserving biodiversity, 160–1

Bangladesh, 31, 100–1, 142, 153, 196
  flood, 173
  Ganges-Brahmaputra delta, 148
Basel Convention on the movement of hazardous waste, 32, 200
basic human needs, inequalities in access to, 30–1
behavioural measures, 114
Beijing Amendment, 157
benzene, 117
Best Practical Environmental Option (BPEO), 75, 209
Bhopal disaster, 173
bias, 82, 209
biodiversity, 41, 140, 160–3, 209
  action on, 165
  food and, 162
  health and, 161–3
biogas, 134
biological environment, 11
biological hazards, 4
  water, 91–100
biological warfare, 180
biomass fuels, 57, 65, 66, 110, 111, 130, 131–5, 209
  indoor air pollution in India, 132–4
  reducing indoor air pollution from, 134–5
black smoke, 118–21
  see also particulates
Blunden, J., 29

Bolivia, 30
bottom-up policy development, 199
Brazil, 30, 189–90
British Medical Association (BMA), 77
Brook, R.D., 112
Brown, L., 67
Brown, P., 73
brown coal, 62
bufo toxins, 162
building design, 124–5
building materials, 124–5
burden of disease
  estimating for air pollution, 118–21
  global burden of environmentally related disease, 6–7
  national burden of disease for India from indoor air pollution, 132–4
Bush, George W., 151
butterfly effect, 156

cadmium, 101
Cairncross, S., 7, 91, 94, 100
campylobacter, 146
Canada, 159
cancer, 63–4, 108, 110, 111
carbon dioxide, 84, 141–2
  forests and, 163–4
carbon monoxide, 108, 110, 116
carbon trading, 152
cardiovascular disease, 108, 110, 111, 112
carrying capacity, 206
Carson, Rachel, 19
cataracts, 158
causality, 133
Central Board of Health, 17
Chagas disease, 144
chemical hazards, 4
  contaminants of water, 100–2
  outdoor air pollution, 108, 109, 110, 111, 116–17

chemical warfare, 179–80
Chen, B., 118
Chernobyl disaster, 58, 63–4
child mortality, 22, 178
children, 130, 174
China, 29, 50, 53, 113, 133, 157
    outdoor air pollution, 114,
        118
    Three Gorges Dam, 61
Chittagong, Bangladesh, 196
chlorofluorocarbons (CFCs), 21,
    141–2, 156, 157
chloroquine, 162
cholera, 93, 145, 146
chromium, 101
chronic exposure, air pollution
    and, 113
cinchona tree, 162
circulatory diseases, 189
Clapp, R., 73
Clean Air Act 1956, 114
Clean Development Mechanism,
    152
climate change, 42–4, 98, 139–55,
    159, 209
    and climate variability, 140–1
    communicable disease and,
        144–7
    effects on human health, 143–4
    environmental movement and,
        19–20
    extreme weather and, 141,
        148–50, 169–71
    global distribution of, 142–3
    origin of greenhouse gases,
        141–2
    physical changes in the
        environment, 148–51
    politics of, 21, 151–4
    and sustainable development,
        152–4
    uncertainties of climate change
        scenarios, 150–1
    waste management and, 84
climate variability, 140–1
climatological events, 168–9, 209
    see also flooding; hurricanes
closed-loop recycling, 76
coal, 132
coal mining industry, 45
cohort studies, 113
cold housing, 126–8
collection of waste, 78, 79
Committee on Health Effects of
    Waste Incineration, 83

Commons, Open Spaces and
    Footpath Preservation Society,
    18
communicable diseases
    and climate change, 144–7
    urban environment, 188
community composting plants, 77
composting, 77, 79, 80, 84
confounding, 82, 209
construction-related problems,
    124–5
consumption, 32, 206
controlled wastes, 70
Convention on Biological
    Diversity, 165
cost
    cost-benefit approach to water
        standards, 103–4
    solid waste management, 79
Côte d'Ivoire, 30
crop yields, 158–9
Cropper, M.L., 113
culture, 14–15, 27, 28
cyanide, 101
Cyclops (water flea), 94

damp housing, 128–9
Darwin, Charles, 18
debt relief, 22
deforestation, 163–5
Delhi, India, 113
dengue/dengue haemorrhagic
    fever, 92, 96, 97, 98, 99,
    145
Denmark, 67
desertification, 140
developing countries *see* low
    income countries
development
    economic, 27, 28, 33–4
    and energy production, 59–60
    equitable, 13, 37, 210
    health, environment and, 3–4
    and spread of vector-borne
        disease, 96–8
    sustainable *see* sustainable
        development
    technological and scientific, 27,
        28, 32–3
    urban environmental issues
        and, 190, 191–2
diarrhoeal diseases, 6–7, 92, 144–6,
    188
difficult wastes, 70
dioxins, 83

disasters, 143, 167–82
    Chernobyl, 58, 63–4
    emergency response and
        planning for, 175–6
    health consequences of war,
        178–81
    man-made, 168, 173–4, 177–8
    management in urban
        environments, 192
    mitigation of, 176–8
    natural, 167, 168–73, 176–7
    psychological effects, 174–5
    responding to disaster, 167–8
disease
    communicable disease and
        climate change, 144–7
    and the environment, 14–15
    transmission of, 17
    urban environment and, 188,
        189
    water, health and, 91–100
diseases of poverty, 188
dispersion of pollutants, 109
dose response relationship, 102
drainage, 191
drinking water, chemicals in, 101
    see also water
driving forces, 26–34, 184, 206,
    209
drugs, 22
    naturally occurring medicines,
        161
D'Souza, C.M., 51

early warning systems, 175–6
Earth-centred perspective, 206
Earth Summit 1992, 8, 20, 151,
    165
earthquakes, 168–9, 176
ecological destruction, 18
ecological footprint, 193–4, 209
ecological vandalism, 180–1
ecology, 13, 209
    pesticides and, 102
economic development, 27, 28,
    33–4
economic infrastructure, 187
economic measures, 114
economic risk, 102–3
economy, 20, 44
ecosystems, 14, 209
    balance of and human health,
        156–66
education, universal primary, 22,
    31

Egypt, 142, 148
EIA, 29
El Niño, 140, 148, 209
electrical and electronic waste, 76
Elliott, P., 82
emergency response planning,
175–6
emissions
greenhouse gases *see* greenhouse
gases
industrial, 45–9, 115
end-of-life vehicles, 76
energy, 56–68
development and energy
production, 59–60
energy efficiency of houses,
128
impacts of energy consumption
on health, 57–8
production and uses of, 57–60
resources, 58–9, 65, 67
and sustainable development,
65–7
use by country groups, 58–9
use and the effect on the
environment, 65
use and environmental
degradation, 60–5
environment, 3, 209
basic requirements for a healthy
environment, 23
changes in due to urbanization,
185–6
current environmental
concerns, 21–3
and development of public
health policies, 15–17
energy use and environmental
degradation, 60–5
health, development and, 3–4
local environment and health,
9–11
physical changes due to climate
change, 148–51
understanding the relationship
between health and the
environment, 14–15
environmental awareness, 18–20
environmental health, 5–6
environmental impact
assessments (EIAs), 165, 201–2
environmental justice, 199, 206,
209
environmental management,
integrating, 51–2

Environmental Protection Agency
(EPA) (US), 20, 199
environmental quality, 41–55
and health, 41–4
industry, 14, 44–52
transport, 4, 50, 52–5, 107,
186
epidemiological studies, 111–12
national burden of disease for
India from indoor air
pollution, 132–4
equitable development, 13, 37,
209
equity, 7–8, 13, 199, 206, 210
climate change and sustainable
development, 152–4
Esrey, S.A., 94
ethanol, 67
ethnicity/race, 31
Europe, 70, 72
see also under individual countries
European Union, 157
air quality standards, 115
eutrophication, 101, 159, 210
excess winter mortality, 126–8
exposure, 13, 35, 210
chronic exposure to air
pollution, 113
environmental exposures and
health, 42–4
routes for waste, 80, 81
extreme weather events, 141,
148–50, 169–71
eyes, damage to, 157–8

Factory Inspectorate, 17
faecal contamination, 91–3, 100
fatal workplace accidents, 46–9
Feachem, R., 91, 100
Fewtrell, L.J., 54
Fiji, 146
filariasis, 92, 96, 98, 99, 144
flooding, 142, 168–9, 172–3
fluoride, 101, 102
food
and biodiversity, 162
polluted, 43–4
refugee/displaced persons
camps, 179
food poisoning, 146
forcing agents, 139, 210
forests, 18, 34, 140, 159, 163–5
formaldehyde, 125
fossil fuels, 57, 107, 110, 111
power generation, 60, 62, 65

Framework Convention on
Climate Change, 151
France, 143, 149
fuel cells, 67
fuel poverty, 128
fungal spores, 129

Ganges-Brahmaputra delta,
Bangladesh, 148
gender equality, 22, 31
General Agreement on Tariffs and
Trade (GATT), 34
genetic modification, 162–3
Geneva Convention, 180
geographical area, 30
geographical information system
(GIS), 144, 210
geological disasters, 168–9,
176
see also tsunamis
germs, 17
Ghana, 189–90
glaciers, 141
Glacken, C., 15
Glasgow, Scotland, 196
global environmental standards,
199
global partnership for
development, 22
global warming *see* climate change
Goa, 85–6
Gosse, P.H., 18
grassroots organizations, 19
grassroots policy, 199
green taxes, 200
greenhouse effect, 140, 141,
142
greenhouse gases, 84, 192, 210
emission targets, 151–2
origin of, 141–2
see also climate change
Greening Industry policy, 50
Greenpeace, 19
Guatemala, 31
guerrilla warfare, 180–1
guinea worm, 93, 94
Gulf War, first, 178, 181
Gupta, A., 18, 59–60, 164, 165,
185, 186

Hague Declaration, 180
Haiti storm, 170–1
harvesting effects, 112
hazardous wastes, 32, 70, 72–3,
77–8, 80, 200

hazards, 26, 34–7, 210
  environmental exposures and
    health, 42–4
  of housing, 125–6
  of the indoor environment,
    123–4
health
  and biodiversity, 161–3
  definition, 5, 210
  differentials and the urban
    environment, 189–90
  effects of air pollutants, 108,
    110–11
  effects of climate change, 143–4
  effects of ozone depletion,
    157–9
  effects of waste disposal, 78–84
  environment, development
    and, 3–4
  environmental impact
    assessments, 201–2
  environmental quality and,
    41–4
  housing and, 124–30
  impacts of energy consumption
    on, 57–8
  inequity by socioeconomic
    group, geographical area,
    gender and race/ethnicity,
    30–1
  relationship between indoor
    environment and, 122–4
  studying the health effects of air
    pollutants, 111–14
  and the urban environment,
    187–90
  water, disease and, 91–100
Healthy Cities programmes,
  194–6, 203
Healthy Islands Project, 204–5
Healthy Villages programmes,
  203–4
heatwaves, 143, 148–50
heavy metals, 83
helminthic infections, 92, 93, 100,
  144
high income cities, 190, 191–2
high income countries, 21, 22, 23
  food poisoning and climate
    change, 146
  hazards of indoor environment,
    124
  solid waste management, 78, 79
  time spent indoors and
    outdoors, 123

waste, 73, 74
high-rise buildings, 125
Hiroshima, Japan, 180
HIV/AIDS, 22
holistic perspective, 206
Home Energy Efficiency Scheme,
  128
hookworm (Necator), 93
hotspots, biodiversity, 160–1
house dust mites, 129
housing, 124–30
  cold housing and excess winter
    mortality, 126–8
  damp housing, 128–9
  design and building materials,
    124–5
  hazards of, 125–6
  over-crowding, 126, 188
  principles of healthy housing,
    129–30
  unhealthy, 43–4
Howden-Chapman, P., 126,
  128
Howe, G.M., 14
human activity, 7, 11
  and the environment, 26–34
  environmental quality and,
    41–55
  health, environment and, 5–6,
    8–9
human-centred perspective, 206
human driving forces, 26–34, 184,
  206, 209
hunger, eradication of, 22, 31
hurricanes, 168–9, 170–1, 176–7
hydrocarbons, 108, 110, 111
hydroelectricity, 60–2, 65, 67
hydrogen, 67
hydrogen sulphide, 116

ice caps, 141
immune system, damage to,
  157–8
incineration, 77, 79, 80, 82–4, 84
India, 31, 50, 94, 113, 157, 165,
  176
  air quality standards, 115–17
  Bhopal disaster, 173
  indoor air pollution, 132–4
  integrating environmental
    management in small
    industries, 51–2
  slums in Mumbai, 186–7
Indonesia, 50
  tsunami, 170, 174

indoor air pollution, 57, 66, 130–5,
  186, 192
  in India, 132–5
  by source, 131
indoor environment, 57, 122–36
  in context, 135
  hazards of, 123–4
  housing and health, 124–30
  low and middle income
    countries, 130–5
  relationship with health,
    122–4
Industrial Revolution, 15–17, 46,
  141, 210
industry, 14, 44–52
  impacts of rapid
    industrialization, 50
  industrial resources and
    emissions, 45–9
  sustainable development and,
    50–2
inequity, 27, 28, 30–1
infectious diseases, 17, 189
information and communication
  technology (ICT), 22, 32–3
infrastructure, 187, 210
integrated waste management
  system, 85–6
integration of policy, 198–200
Intergovernmental Panel on
  Climate Change (IPCC), 140,
  141, 153
Intermediate Technology
  Development Group, 33
international assistance, 174–5
international cooperation, 20–3
  on climate change, 21, 151–2
  current environmental
    concerns, 21–3
  policy making, 200–2
International Labour Organization
  (ILO), 49
inter-sectoral collaboration,
  200–1, 202–5, 210
intestinal nematodes, 92, 93, 100,
  144
invermectin, 96
Iran, 50, 203, 204
Iraq, 178
Ireland, 162

Jamaica, 186
Japan, 180
Japanese encephalitis, 98
job security, 200

Johannesburg summit, 23, 160, 165

Katsouyanni, K., 112
Kawata, K., 92
Keats, John, 18
kerosene, 66
Kingston, Jamaica, 186
Koch, Robert, 17
Kovats, R.S., 153
Kuching, Malaysia, 195
Kunzli, N., 113
Kyoto Protocol, 67, 151–2, 200
Kyrgyzstan, 48, 49

laboratory studies, 111
land management, 192
landfill, 77, 78, 79, 80–2, 84, 210
landfill taxes, 74–5
landmines, 180–1
Landon, M., 50
Last, A., 35
lead, 53–4, 108, 110, 117
lifestyle, 18, 188
local community committees, 203–4
local emergency plans, 175
local standards, 200
London
    air pollution and daily mortality, 118–21
    smog of December 1952, 111
London Declaration on Action in Partnership, 201
long-term (chronic) effects, 112–13
Lopez, A., 54
Love Canal, 72–3
low income cities, 191–2
low income countries, 9, 21, 22, 23
    air quality management, 118
    hazards of indoor environment, 124
    indoor air pollution, 130–5
    solid waste management, 78, 79
    time spent indoors and outdoors, 123
    waste, 73, 74
    waste picking, 84–6
lower-middle income cities, 191–2
lyme disease, 144

maize, 162

malaria, 22
    climate change and, 145, 146–7
    modelling the distribution of, 147
    and quinine, 162
    Solomon Islands Project, 204–5
    water, health and disease, 92, 94–6, 98, 99
Malaysia, 195
Maldives, 148
malnutrition, 133
man-made disasters, 168, 173–4
    mitigation of, 177–8
    see also war
Manchester, UK, 159
Markandya, A., 64
Marshall Islands, 142, 148
maternal health, 22
McGranahan, G., 190
McMichael, A.J., 113, 142, 157, 159, 161, 162, 184, 193, 206
Medical Officer of Health, 17
melanoma, 158
meningococcal meningitis, 145
Menne, B., 64
mercury, 101
methane, 84, 141–2
methyl-isocyanate, 173
Mexico, 30
Mexico City, 107
miasmas, 17
microfinance, 33–4
middle income cities, 191–2
middle income countries, 21
    air quality management, 118
    hazards of indoor environment, 124
    indoor air pollution, 130–5
    solid waste management, 78, 79
    time spent indoors and outdoors, 123
    waste, 73, 74
    waste picking, 84–6
migration, 186
Millennium Declaration, 21, 31, 200
Millennium Development Goals (MDGs), 21–3, 31, 59, 163, 205, 206
Millennium Ecosystem Assessment, 165
modelling
    climate change, 141, 150–1
    distribution of malaria, 147
modern hazards, 35–6, 123–4

Moeller, D.W., 58, 169, 175–6
Molina, M., 157
Montreal Protocol, 157
mortality, 9
    air pollution and daily mortality in London, 118–21
    child mortality, 22, 178
    cold housing and excess winter mortality, 126–8
    due to European heatwave 2003, 149
    time-series studies of air pollution and, 112
mortality displacement (harvesting), 112
mould, 128–9
Mozambique, 180–1
Muir, John, 18
multilateral trade agreements/negotiations, 34
Mumbai, India, 186–7
Murray, C., 54

Nabuel, Tunisia, 195–6
Nagasaki, Japan, 180
national emergency plans, 175
national policy, 200
natural disasters, 167, 168–73
    mitigation of, 176–7
natural sciences, 18
naturally-occurring medicines, 161
nematodes (worms), 92, 93, 100, 144
Netherlands, the, 142
New Zealand, 175, 176
Ngubane, H., 14–15
Nigeria, 30
Nile delta, Egypt, 148
nitrates, 101
nitrogen dioxide, 108, 109, 118–19
nitrogen monoxide, 108
nitrogen oxides, 108, 110, 116, 141–2, 159–60
no acceptable risk approach, 102
no excess risk approach, 102
non-governmental organizations (NGOs), 19
non-renewable energy resources, 58, 65
Nordhaus, T., 20
nuclear fuel cycle, 64–5
nuclear power, 58, 60, 63–4
nuclear warfare, 180

Nuon, 152
nutrients, 101

occupational accidents, 46–9
onchocerciasis, 96, 99
open fires, 131–2
open-loop recycling, 76
'Ordinaryville', 9–11
outdoor air pollution, 42–4,
    105–21, 192
  air quality, 114–18
  energy use and, 57, 60, 62
  estimating burden of disease
    resulting from air pollution,
    118–21
  industrial pollution, 46
  and public health, 106–11
  sources of air pollution, 106–8
  studying health effects of
    pollutants, 111–14
  transport and, 52, 53–4
  types of air pollution, 108–11
  waste disposal and, 83–4
over-crowding, 126, 188
ozone, 108, 109, 111, 116, 118–19,
    159–60
ozone layer depletion, 21, 140,
    156–9, 211

Pacific islands, 148, 153
Pacific yew, 162
Packaging Regulations, 74–5
packaging waste, 76
Pakistan, 31, 94
Panaji waste management system,
    85–6
parasitic diseases, 189
particulates, 210
  indoor air pollution 132, 133,
    134–5
  outdoor air pollution, 83, 106–8,
    108, 110, 111, 116, 118–21
Pasteur, Louis, 17
patient characteristics, 106, 210
Patz, J.A., 153
Peat, J.K., 129
penicillin, 161
Periès, H., 94
peri-urban areas, 88, 193, 210
Peru, 30, 33, 146
pesticides, 101–2
petroleum products, 65, 66
Philippines, 50
phosphates, 101
photochemical oxidants, 108, 110

photochemical smog, 108, 109,
    111, 210
photokeratitis, 158
physical environment, 11, 188
physical hazards, 4
physical measures, 114
phytoplankton, 159
planning
  for disasters, 175–6
  for a healthy city, 194–6
plant breeding, 162
plants, 158–9
policy, 198–207
  Agenda 21, 20, 200–1, 202–5
  development of public health
    policies, 15–17
  integration for environmental
    health and sustainable
    development, 198–200
  international policy making,
    200–2
  national policy, 200
  sustainable future, 205–6
poliomyelitis, 92
political systems, 27, 28
polycyclic aromatic hydrocarbons
    (PAHs), 102
Poor Law Amendment Act 1834,
    16
Poor Law Commission, 16–17
Pope, C., 20, 113
population, 27, 28, 28–30, 32
population studies see
    epidemiological studies
potato famine, 162
poverty
  diseases of, 188
  eradication of, 22, 31, 206
  and inequity, 27, 28, 30–1
  urban environment, 186,
    189–90
power generation, 60–5
precautionary principle, 17, 157,
    206, 210
pre-event phase, 175, 177
primary education, universal, 22
primary pollutants, 109, 210
primary recycling, 76
processed fuels, 134
production
  capitalist and Industrial
    Revolution, 15
  global increase in, 21
protection from sea-level rise, 148
proximity principle, 75, 84

psychological effects
  of disasters, 174–5
  of over-crowding, 126
  of urban environment, 185,
    188–9
public concern, 71–3
public disclosure programme, 50
public health
  environment and development
    of public health policies,
    15–17
  outdoor air pollution and,
    106–11
Public Health Act 1848, 17
pulmonary disease, 130

quinine, 162

race/ethnicity, 31
radionuclides, 63, 210
radon, 125
rainfall, 143
rapid industrialization, 50
recovery/rehabilitation phase,
    176, 177
recycling, 76–7, 79
reduction of waste, 74–5, 75–6, 79
refugees, 178–9
regional emergency plans, 175
rehabilitation/recovery phase,
    176, 177
relative risk, 56, 210
remote sensing, 144, 210
renewable energy resources, 58,
    65
  and sustainable development,
    67
resources, industrial, 45–9
respiratory diseases, 7
  indoor environment, 129, 130
  outdoor air pollution, 108, 110,
    111
  urban environment, 188, 189
response phase, 176, 177
retreat strategy, 148
re-use, 76–7
rice, 162
Rift Valley fever, 145
Rio Earth Summit, 8, 20, 151, 165
risk mapping, 144
risk transition, 4, 14, 36–7, 190,
    211
risks, 26, 34–7, 211
river blindness (onchocerciasis),
    96, 99

road transport, 4, 50, 52–5, 107, 186
Romanticism, 18
Ross River virus, 145
roundworm (*Ascaris*), 93
Rowland, F.S., 157
Russia, 151

salmonella, 146
sanitation, 99–100, 191, 204–5
  Victorian era, 15–17
São Paulo, Brazil, 189–90
sarin, 180
Sarre, P., 29
Satterthwaite, D., 194–5, 195–6
Saudi Arabia, 115–17
Scandinavia, 159
scenarios, climate change, 150–1
Schiller, J.C.F., 18
schistosomiasis, 92, 93–4, 98, 144
Schwela, D., 123
scientific development, 27, 28, 32–3
Scotland, 196
sea-level rise, 141, 148, 153
secondary pollutants, 109, 211
secondary recycling, 76
sectors, waste generation by, 70–1, 72
selenium, 101
Selvam, P., 85–6
Senegal, 96
sewage, 99–100
  see also sanitation
Shell, 152
Shellenberger, M., 20
Sierra Club, 18, 19
sievert, 56, 211
Singh, R.B.K., 146
skin cancer, 157–8
slums, 186–7
small-scale industry, 46–9
  environmental management in India, 51–2
Smith, K.R., 113, 132–3
smog, 107, 109, 114, 211
  photochemical, 108, 109, 111, 210
socioeconomic differentiation, 186–7, 211
socioeconomic environment, 188
socioeconomic group, 30
soil pollution, 46, 60
solid fuels, 65, 130, 132

solid wastes
  management in different countries, 78, 79
  sources, 70, 71
  see also waste
Solomon Islands Healthy Islands Project, 204–5
South Africa, 31
South-East Asian tsunami, 167, 169–70, 174, 175
squatter settlements, 186–7
Sri Lanka, 170
standards
  air quality, 114–17
  global environmental standards, 199
  local, 200
  setting for water supply quality, 102–4
Stockholm Declaration 1972, 20
stoves, 132, 134
Strategic Environmental Assessment (SEA) Protocol, 201–2
stratospheric ozone depletion, 21, 140, 156–9, 211
Sub-Saharan Africa, 94
subsidies, 200
sulphur, 116
sulphur dioxide, 108, 109, 110, 118–19, 159
sulphur oxides, 110, 111
surface temperature rise, 141, 148
Sustainable Cities movement, 203
sustainable development, 4, 7–8, 20, 23–4, 211
  climate change and, 152–4
  and energy use, 59, 65–7
  environment, health and, 3–4
  and industry, 50–2
  Millennium Development Goal, 22, 31
  renewable energy and, 67
  tropical forests, 164–5
  urbanization and, 190–4
system failure, 149

Tanzania, 4
targets, for greenhouse gas emissions, 151–2
task forces, 195
taxol, 162
technological development, 27, 28, 32–3

technology transfer, 32
terrorism, 180–1
Thailand, 50
Thérivel, R., 201
Three Gorges Dam, 61
time
  and access to water, 90–1
  spent indoors and outdoors, 122, 123
  spent looking for wood, 132
time-series analysis, 111–13
  air pollution and daily mortality in London, 118–21
top-down policy development, 198–9
Torrey Canyon, 19
toxic chemicals, 159
trachoma, 92, 93
trade, 22, 34
traditional hazards, 35–6, 123–4
transport, 4, 50, 52–5, 107, 186
  and accidents, 54
  and air pollution, 52, 53–4
  of wastes, 84
trees
  benefits of urban trees, 193–4
  see also forests
trisect of sustainable business, 51
Tropical Forest Action Plan (TFAP), 165
tropical forests, 34, 163–5
tropical storms, 170–1, 172
tsunamis, 167, 168–9, 169–70, 174, 211
Tunisia, 195–6
tyres, used, 80–2

ultraviolet (UV) radiation, 156–9, 211
UNCED, 8
uncertainty, 150–1
UNDP, 132
UNEP, 157
UNFPA, 28, 31, 32
Union Carbide, 173
United Kingdom (UK), 4, 18, 114, 115, 159
  air quality standards, 115–17
  development of public health policies, 15–17
  outdoor air pollution, 106–8
  waste management strategy, 75
  winter excess mortality, 126–8

United Nations (UN), 5, 163, 175, 200
  Millennium Development Goals, 21–3, 31, 59, 163, 205, 206
United Nations Conference on the Human Environment (Earth Summit), 8, 20, 151, 165
United Nations Framework Convention on Climate Change, 151
United Nations Millennium Summit, 21
United States (USA), 151, 152, 157
  environmental awareness, 18, 20
  EPA, 20, 199
  Love Canal, 72–3
  waste production, 73
Universal Declaration of Human Rights, 8
upper-middle income cities, 191–2
uranium, 101
uranium mining, 63
urban environment, 109, 183–97, 211
  defining, 184–5
  economic infrastructure, 185, 187
  environmental risk transition, 190
  health and, 187–90
  impacts of rapid industrialization, 50
  issues and development, 190, 191–2
  modifying the natural environment for urbanization, 185–6
  physical aspects, 185, 186
  planning for a healthy city, 194–6
  psychosocial aspects, 185, 188
  social and cultural aspects, 185, 186–7
  urbanization as driving force, 27, 28, 28–30
  urbanization and sustainable development, 190–4

vector-borne diseases
  environmental factors in the spread of, 96–9
  water-related, 92, 94–9
vectors, 17, 211

ventilation, 131
Vienna Convention, 157
Vietnam, 50
Vietnam War, 180
volatile organic compounds, 160
volcanic eruptions, 168–9

war, 178–81
  direct environmental effects, 179–81
  indirect environmental effects, 178–9
warning/alerting phase, 175–6, 177
waste, 42–4, 46, 69–87
  disposal in refugee/displaced persons camps, 179
  global issues of waste management, 84–6
  hazardous, 32, 70, 72–3, 77–8, 80, 200
  health effects of waste disposal, 78–84
  improving final disposal and monitoring, 77
  management, 73–8, 191
  prevention/minimization, 74–5, 75–6, 79
  public concern, 71–3
  quantifying, 73, 74
  recycling, 76–7, 79
  re-use, 76–7
  solid waste management in different countries, 78, 79
  Solomon Islands Project, 204–5
  sources, 70–1, 72
  urban environment and, 193
waste hierarchy, 73–5, 211
waste picking, 84–6
water, 88–105, 133, 140
  access to, 89–91
  chemical contaminants, 100–2
  health, disease and, 91–100
  pollution, 42–4, 46, 100–2
  power generation and water pollution, 60
  recycling of waste water, 77
  standard-setting for quality of the water supply, 102–4
  supply in refugee/displaced persons camps, 179
  supply and the urban environment, 191
  unsafe and climate change, 144–6

uses and quality required, 89–90
Victorian era, 15–17
water engineer's dilemma, 103–4
water-based disease, 92, 93–4, 211
water-borne disease, 91–3, 211
water-related vector-borne diseases, 92, 94–9, 211
  prevention, 98–9
water scarcity, 89, 211
water-washed disease, 92, 93, 211
wheat, 162
whipworm (*Trichuris*), 93
Whitelegg, J., 53
Wilkinson, P., 126–8
wind power, 67
winter excess mortality, 126–8
women, 9, 91, 130
  empowerment of, 22, 31
wood-burning stoves, 132
wood fuel *see* biomass fuels
Wordsworth, William, 18
workplace injuries, fatal, 46–9
World Bank, 50, 71, 130
World Commission on Environment and Development, 7
World Health Organization (WHO), 95, 100
  air quality standards, 115–17
  basic requirements for a healthy environment, 23
  communicable disease and climate change, 144, 145
  definition of health, 5
  guidelines for inorganic chemicals in drinking water, 101
  Healthy Cities initiative, 194–6
  healthy living through sustainable development, 24
  Healthy Villages programme, 203–4
  inequity in health by socioeconomic group, geographical area, gender and race/ethnicity, 30–1
  principles of healthy housing, 129–30
  psychological effects of disasters, 174
  risk transition, 36–7
  Solomon Islands Project, 204–5
  strategies for adaptation to sea-level rise, 148

World Health Report, 92
World Summit on Sustainable
    Development (Johannesburg,
    2002), 23, 160, 165
World Trade Centre terrorist
    attacks, 181

World Trade Organization (WTO),
    34
worms, 92, 93, 100, 144

Yassi, A., 160, 168
yellow fever, 96, 99

Yosemite National Park,
    18

Zimbabwe, 33–4
zooplankton, 159
Zulus, 14–15

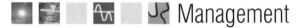
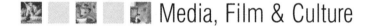
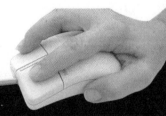